The
Silver Branch
and the
Otherworld

"Not just an important contribution to herbal medicine, but a significant contribution to Irish literature itself."

MATTHEW WOOD, HERBALIST AND AUTHOR OF
A SHAMANIC HERBAL

"Herbalist and poet Seán Pádraig O'Donoghue weaves together the enchantment of Celtic and personal history, emotions, physiology, herbal wisdom, and therapeutic insights with profound interpretations. You'll learn from his favorite authors as well as the herbs, trees, fungi, and friends imparted through his unique sensory experiences. Encounters with animals, the moon and stars, the glowing sun, and the elements flow through the pages of this book like a wild stream. This becomes a visceral adventure filled with original insights, meditations, and rituals designed to reconnect us to a nature-based life. *The Silver Branch and the Otherworld* invites readers to breathe deeply and reengage with our world."

MARGI FLINT, RH, HM,
AUTHOR OF *THE PRACTICING HERBALIST*

"Seán Pádraig O'Donoghue lives as well as dreams this quest-full story that his books and classes tell—intensely, tragically, joyously, and epically. *The Silver Branch and the Otherworld* serves as a portal into the expressive magic of what is the real and true world, a path leading the reader toward self-understanding and personalized purpose as well as to the profound healings and revelations of the plants found there. It is my pleasure to encourage his continuing sharings, songs of determination, and hopes for you as you enter into the chiaroscuro light of enchanted forests and Druid's groves."

JESSE WOLF HARDIN, ARTIST AND
AUTHOR OF *FUNGI MEDICA* AND *THE HERBALIST*

"When I first step into the forest, my cathedral, I am overwhelmed by the quiet and the awareness that 'much silence has a mighty roar.' And when I read Seán's poetic vision, breathing life into the wisdom of our plant and fungal allies, I am reminded of a connection that vibrates so deeply, so powerfully, that I am moved to tears, joy, and wonderment all at the same time."

ROBERT DALE ROGERS, HERBALIST AND AUTHOR OF
MEDICINAL LICHENS: INDIGENOUS WISDOM AND MODERN PHARMACOLOGY

"There has always been a gentleness and deep embodiment in Seán's writing. Like a forest laughing or a stone singing, every part of this book will speak to you in a voice not just heard, but also felt—and this is how we best come to learn what is true."

RHYD WILDERMUTH, DRUID AND AUTHOR OF
BEING PAGAN: A GUIDE TO RE-ENCHANT YOUR LIFE

"Seán speaks to the heart of those of us in the Irish diaspora who long to connect with ancestral wisdom even as we seek to root into the land we now call home. Weaving myth and scientific knowledge, poetry and a palpable sense of reverence, *The Silver Branch and the Otherworld* invites you to come home to yourself, your spiritual lineage, and your own wild kin."

MARISA GOUDY, HOST OF *KNOTWORK STORYTELLING*
AND AUTHOR OF *THE SOVEREIGNTY KNOT*

"This book is an antidote to the long loneliness of the human species. In a world out of balance, it serves as a balm to the agitated spirit and offers a map for navigating the territory of changes the Earth and all members of the ecological community are currently experiencing. *The Silver Branch and the Otherworld* is a much-needed guide and manifesto of hope for navigating these troubling times through the power of story. It reminds us of our deeply rooted connections to the Green world and the world of myth and legend, reaffirming that we are not alone."

JULIE MCINTYRE, EARTH CEREMONIALIST, DIRECTOR OF THE
CENTER FOR EARTH RELATIONS, AND AUTHOR OF
SEX AND THE INTELLIGENCE OF THE HEART

The
Silver Branch
and the
Otherworld

Forest Magic
with Plant and Fungi Allies

A Sacred Planet Book

Seán Pádraig O'Donoghue

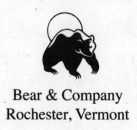

Bear & Company
Rochester, Vermont

Bear & Company
One Park Street
Rochester, Vermont 05767
www.BearandCompanyBooks.com

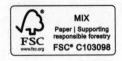

Bear & Company is a division of Inner Traditions International

Sacred Planet Books are curated by Richard Grossinger, Inner Traditions editorial board member and cofounder and former publisher of North Atlantic Books. The Sacred Planet collection, published under the umbrella of the Inner Traditions family of imprints, includes works on the themes of consciousness, cosmology, alternative medicine, dreams, climate, permaculture, alchemy, shamanic studies, oracles, astrology, crystals, hyperobjects, locutions, and subtle bodies.

Cataloging-in-Publication Data for this title is available from the Library of Congress

ISBN 978-1-59143-472-6 (print)
ISBN 978-1-59143-473-3 (ebook)

Printed and bound in the United States by Lake Book Manufacturing, LLC

10 9 8 7 6 5 4 3 2 1

Text design and layout by Kenleigh Manseau
This book was typeset in Garamond Premier Pro with Steagal Roughused as a display typeface

To send correspondence to the author of this book, mail a first-class letter to the author c/o Inner Traditions • Bear & Company, One Park Street, Rochester, VT 05767, and we will forward the communication, or contact the author directly at **otherworldwell.com**.

Scan the QR code and save 25% at InnerTraditions.com.
Browse over 2,000 titles on spirituality, the occult, ancient mysteries, new science, holistic health, and natural medicine.

for
Mo Bhanríon Fiáin agus Mo Sionnach Beag
with deep gratitude for
the braiding of the wild roads we walk

and in loving memory of
Stephen Harrod Buhner

Contents

The Forest Reminds Us Who We Are

Dr. Mitchell Bebel Stargrove

Entering a book, an unimagined yet somehow clear perception opens, and a sense of familiar experience arises. The objective and subjective flow back and forth into each other as past memory, immediate sensation, and future visions reveal patterns of emergence grounded in knowing within relationship.

After many years of observing Seán in his glories and travails, I see here a story of a storyteller being told. He shares synchronicities and revelations while weaving history, poetry, plants, and life sciences throughout the events and relationships of his experience. As Seán has matured in his storytelling, he has achieved a dynamic equilibrium between oral tradition and written presentation. The expanded openness that Seán generates when speaking is accessed and induced by these words of magick.

Having known Seán for many years, I've often felt a shared comfort and discomfort with Seán, a vague sense of familiarity, of us being revolutionaries together or, more poignantly, two heretical Catholic priests of long ago, an Irishman and a Pole, pondering more ancient memories in involuntary seclusion. We found ourselves natural allies engaged in social medicine and applied natural therapies toward creating regenerative cultures and birthing a new aeon every day. Loving the ancient past, especially before empire, Seán reveals visions and shares deeply felt experiences that are the daily reality of our process of cocreating healthy futures in alignment with Gaia. Rooted in our ancestors, honoring the lands in which we live, and manifesting the art of living, together—this is the work of these times.

The presence, tone, and voice of this book are vividly Seán's, as reflected in his approach and improvisation, and this extends to the content itself. The working vision framing this book is rooted in an ancient three-worlds model and expands into ecology, complexity theory, bioregional reintegration, and postbinary culture. Seán thrives on igniting enthusiasm in each of us as he demonstrates that science can be mythic and that the mythic is immediate and omnipresent. This is more than an herb book because in it we experience plant medicine through relationships and observations of living networks. While proudly identifying as neurodivergent, Seán makes no claim to exclusive access to hidden secrets. He serves as a poet, storyteller, and guide, as well as a Gaian herbalist modeling mythically informed embodied awareness as a postbinary visionary activist.

Seán is an exemplar of a modern successor to the Draoi of pre-Christian Ireland, weaving magick and science, poetry and physiology with plants and charms, thus creating radical possibilities. As Carl Jung exhorts, learning the traditions of other cultures can enrich us, but we gain power and insight from aligning with the deep roots of our own heritages, particularly, in this case, the folk traditions of Europe. Known by specific indigenous names in each culture, they are distinguished by initiated lineages, offer a panoply of medicine and magick, and are the ones who provided medical care for most folks throughout history. Looking back, it becomes all too evident that there is a big hole in our medical history. If classical physicians of the past were treating only the elites, who was providing medical care for most of the population, especially in the rural areas, hamlets, and small towns where most people lived? Hidden between the "educated" physicians and the unnamed of family self-care, they would gather and prescribe herbs, use enchanted psalms, counsel with astrology and divination, clear curses, invoke mates, and help with a variety of problems of family, home, and farm.

I smile when I see the excitement of discovery in the eyes of students and practitioners of natural medicine about the nonphysician lineages of medical practice in premodern Europe. They often say that they feel reconnected to a deep part of their own history and to medicine's pos-sibilities, which embody long-lost "relatives of blood and bone, of vision and service." I see many who aspire to a profession that draws from both the classical physician and the mythic witch-shaman, as well as from the old wives and medicine people. They do so to express an authentic con-temporary synthesis realized in moments of synchronistic certainty but, as yet, not fully imagined. In this work, Seán demonstrates that this can be done, playing upon the emerging edge where the outer intervention of medicine dances with the inner art of self-healing.

> *Seán goes deep. Seán soars.*
> *Seán suffers. Seán celebrates.*
> *Seán smiles silently in bliss.*
> *Seán is a Heathen,*
> *Fear Feasa,*
> *Witch,*
> *WortCharmer,*
> *Cunning Man,*
> *Bard and—*
> *rEvolutionary.*

If you seek a natural-therapies recipe book to see what you might take for your headache, gut pain, or insomnia, in this book you may find exactly what you need, yet maybe not in the way you expected.

However, once you have shared some space-time with Seán and his words, you may never feel the same way as you walk through the forest and fields. Many books offer knowledge in what medicine does, but only a few show us how healing is catalyzed, the transformation that can happen born through experience and deep relationship with plants.

Whether inviting Devil's Club or Damiana, mycelial interplay or Bear magick—or offering a juicy poem or gem of physiology—Seán moves the dance into unexplored perceptual territory embodying mysteries. Yet the wisdom shared here is of a journey taken together, even if we each experience completely different plants, places, or events as we read. Seán activates the reader as if through gnostic *shaktipat,* spreading seeds of spontaneous recognition and offering medicine for each and all. Revealing his deepest aspirations for and dedication to healing, justice, and peace, Seán challenges himself and the reader to fully engage in the experiment of socially conscious compassionate engagement. This experiment embodies manifesting Gandhian self-reliance, mutual aid ethics, and heathen embodiments on the edge of civilization.

Seán is a permissionary, reminding us that we always have permission to be true to our self-knowing and self-creating. He invites us into experiential gnostic learning by telling us to just take a few drops daily and see, feel, and heal. As befits a skillful *satyagraha* truth-force warrior, Seán enters our world by invitation, catalyzes a latent potency toward self-healing and reorganization, and, smiling, silently steps aside as the emergent process unfolds. The method and content of his transmissions remind us to stay attuned to the mythopoetic wellspring of our deep being. This is the source of healing, connection, and renewal. Healing is not primarily about medicine or herbs or even about symptoms improving; rather, healing comes as we deepen our perception, transform our experience, and come to peace with life as it is.

All medicine ultimately relies on self-healing, and in these times, we are healing within ourselves and in our relationships and behaviors as we align with Gaia, of which we are all part. The coherent life flow moving through this planet as a dynamic living system is the same as the vitality and self-organizing processes within our bodies. The metaphor and the biology overlap and enrich each other. This is the rich forest into which we venture with Seán, through many eras and at many scales of becoming.

To quote Seán, "deepening of awareness is a fundamental part of the healing process."

Healing ripples long after medicine treats. This book teaches and activates the reader on all levels, nourishing the root, connecting information through relationships and patterns, and inspiring the heart-mind. As with any journey, the experiences along the way enrich life afterward.

ENJOY, AND
BE WELL,
DR. MITCH STARGROVE

Mitchell Bebel Stargrove, N.D., LAc, earned degrees in acupuncture and naturopathy from Oregon College of Oriental Medicine and the National College of Naturopathic Medicine. He is licensed as an acupuncturist and naturopathic physician in Oregon and practices with Lori Beth Stargrove, N.D., at A WellSpring of Natural Health, in Beaverton. Stargrove is the developer and editor in chief of Integrative BodyMind Information System (IBIS), an encyclopedic reference work of natural medicine, and editor and coauthor of *Herb, Nutrient, and Drug Interactions: Clinical Implications and Therapeutic Strategies* (Mosby, 2008).

FOREWORD TO THE NEW EDITION

The Silver Branch and the Otherworld

Cornelia Benavidez

Books are worthwhile when they are entertaining and certainly earn bonus points when they are educational, yet it is rare when a writer gives as genuinely and richly as Seán does in his book *The Silver Branch*. This should not be a surprise to me because I have had the honor and privilege of being Seán's teacher in the Victor Anderson Feri Tradition, as well as in the Crossroad Tradition, which was taught to me by a woman who was also a wonderful poet (as was Victor), Margaret Korwin DePonzi.

I have never been listened too so intently, so well, or been as honestly engaged with as I was and am with Seán. It is such a joy when a student asks well-thought-out questions as both of us dug deep into the history of what it means to dedicate oneself to an ancient path of wonder, meaning, and challenge.

Why do I use the word *ancient*? Because Seán intuitively understood that our Craft is a path of the earliest service and always has been historically so. He artfully wove together his many skills, and like the plants Seán so dearly loves, he immersed and emerged with regained awareness of the profound gifts of the natural world. To live with such willing openness takes great love and courage, especially when one is willing to talk and walk your experiences to the world as authentically as Seán does.

Herbal wisdom and the healing arts have been with us for hundreds of thousands of years. They show up not only in oral and written lore but also in our most sacred writings from the world over in every culture and religion. The work and roles of the shaman, medicine person, midwife, mystical healer, and priest or priestess historically can be intertwined or separate depending on culture. Those who were and are called to the path to heal physical, emotional, and mental wounds and appeal to the spirit world.

To undertake such work in modern times is not easy and can be tricky as well as dangerous. Why? you might ask. Because rigorous and honest self-reflection on one's soul and spiritual growth to assess one's place in the world is never easy, especially when you are asked to leave behind all that you assume to be true.

In this book, you get an honest, fair, and balanced taste of what it means to awake to wisdom and your true self, as well as the deep powers of the nature, through the herbal world. For Seán it means to be a healer, a poet, a philosopher, a teacher, and a priest, sovereign to and with the land, in order to help show us a deeper and richer way of being.

CORNELIA BENAVIDEZ

Cornelia Benavidez graduated from Albion College, majoring in philosophy, theater, and psychology. She is the author of three books: *Victor Anderson: An American Shaman* (Megalilthic Books, 2017), *Transpiration: Poetry & Storytelling as Our Spiritual Portals* (Megalilthic Books, 2018), and *Journey for a Tomorrow* (Megalilthic Books, 2019). Benavidez has written for *Punk Globe Magazine* and also writes fantasy under the name C. B. Doyle. She is the cofounder, along with her husband, John Doyle, of H.E.A.R. (Hearing, Education and Awareness for Rockers). They live in Oregon, where she continues to write and practice her Craft.

PREFACE

The Life of This Book

A book has a life of its own.

Several years ago, I set out to write what I expected to be a book about the intersections of herbalism, ecopsychology, and somatics. But ancestral voices and stories insisted on weaving themselves in and changing the nature of the book, which began to move in new directions. I let them find their way into the text, but I kept trying to rein them in and write the relatively conventional clinical herbal manual I had promised. That book, *The Forest Reminds Us Who We Are*, had its own brief life in the world, and I am grateful that it found its way to many who could sense the message at the heart of it.

This book, *The Silver Branch*, is, in many ways, what *The Forest Reminds Us Who We Are* would have been had I allowed the spirit of the book to find its own true expression. Parts of that first book have found new life here.

The Silver Branch is an expression of my own practice of cultivating a living practice born of seeds and roots of Irish animist traditions in North American soil. This is not an attempt at reconstructing ancient practices or at transplanting or translating the contemporary Irish practices that grow from these same roots and seeds. It is, rather, a way of giving the gifts of my ancestors new life in another time and place.

There are scholars of history and archaeology and anthropology and Gaeilge literature whose work I love and admire. I am none of these things. I am a poet, an herbalist, and a priest.

Archaeology and anthropology, ethnography and literary scholarship can tell us much about the relationships the people of a particular time and place have or had with gods, animals, plants, mountains, rivers, stars, and oceans. But they do not offer the last word on the nature of our other-than-human kin.

While I reference and draw on old stories and ancestral ways, my writing ultimately arises from my own relationships with the beings of this world and the Otherworld.

Acknowledgments

I give thanks first of all to the plants, the land, the water, and my ancestors, human and wild, and then to my Beloved, who encouraged and inspired me throughout its writing.

Stephen Harrod Buhner, who died while I was completing this book, was a friend, a teacher, and an inspiration. He taught me how to listen directly to the voices of the plants and how to live, speak, and write from my heart. He was also an important force in bringing this book into the world.

My dear friend and teacher Cornelia Benavidez (and her husband, John Doyle) pored over many drafts of this manuscript, offering a keen eye and wonderful suggestions and insights. She is also a deep well of wisdom and inspiration and my living connection to her teachers, Victor and Cora Anderson, whose work and teachings, along with Cornelia's own, have transformed my life in such beautiful and profound ways, though I never met Victor and Cora while they were alive.

My mother, Sandy Donahue, helped to edit some of the early drafts of some of the material in this book. She also introduced me to poetry, myth, and folklore and fed me my first wild foods. My father, Brian Donahue, taught me who the O'Donoghues were and are and taught me to be proud of my Irish ancestry. He and my brother, Ryan, and my sister, Shannon, have been wonderfully encouraging throughout this process.

Crystal Murphy and Denny Sargent helped to edit earlier versions of this book. Michelle Hindman offered her considerable editing skills to the final phases of this it. A host of friends helped me hunt down citations.

Alicia Crockett believed in this book and in me even when I didn't. Thank you.

Many of the ideas that gave rise to this book found their earliest expression in articles I wrote for *Plant Healer* magazine and at the conferences organized by its editors, Kiva Rose Hardin, and Jesse Wolf Hardin. I am deeply grateful for the kindness, inspiration, and insight they have both provided over the years and for their deep commitment to the healing and reenchantment of the world.

Dr. Mitch Bebel Stargrove and Dr. Lori Stargrove shared many nights of conversation with me around their kitchen table, with other eclectic thinkers sometimes joining us. These conversations echo through parts of this book.

Sage Maurer helped me find my way to Ireland and introduced me to its sacred wells, and Alan Cooke helped me connect more deeply with the spirit of the land and introduced me to the work of John Moriarty.

Dr. Kenneth Proefrock's lectures helped me rediscover my childhood love of science and understand neurochemistry and phytochemistry and their implications for consciousness.

Nick Walker's writing about neurodiversity, neurodivergence, and the Autistic mind and experience helped me understand my own neurobiology.

I have learned so much about the lives and medicine of wild plants from so many herbalists over the years. I am grateful to everyone who has ever sat with me and spoke about plants. There are three herbalists whose guidance I especially want to give thanks for:

Margi Flint taught me how to read the body and how to meet people where they are and walk with them on their healing journeys.

Matthew Wood taught me how to read energetic patterns and how to understand the unique medicine and personality of each plant.

Mischa Schuler introduced me to herbalism.

All three of them have shown tremendous kindness and generosity in good times and hard times and have my endless gratitude.

Thank you, finally, to Richard Grossinger, Renée Heitman, Kate Mueller, and everyone at Inner Traditions whose dedicated work helped this book find its way into your hands.

Go raibh maith agaibh.

And see ye not that bonny road
That winds about the fernie brae?
That is the road to fair Elfland
Where thou and I this night maun gae

CHILD BALLAD 37, "THOMAS RHYMER"

Beyond the Walls of Perception

The wooded swamp behind my parents' house was my sanctuary as a child.

Though I was born to a loving family, I never felt at home in my body or in the world. My thoughts and perceptions seemed out of synch with those of everyone around me. Though language held beauty and pleasure for me, ordinary speech never seemed able to bridge the gap between what I was feeling and what the people around me could understand. Poetry became the only accurate way of giving language to my inner experience.

A century earlier I might have been called a changeling. A decade or so later, the many specialists I was sent to might have correctly understood that I was Autistic. Growing up in Massachusetts through the late 1970s and the 1980s, I was simply a sensitive, precocious child with a strange ability to grasp things beyond my peers' or elders' ken and a strange inability to tie my shoes or follow a set of linear instructions.

Like many children, I grew up knowing viscerally that the world was alive. Being Autistic, I held onto that knowledge longer than most people do in this culture.

Autistic brains create more synapses than other brains, and those synapses proliferate in nonlinear ways. Hence, our brains are likely to observe patterns and connections that others miss—and rebel against accepting structures that do not conform to our experience of reality. We also take in more sensory information than most people, which can be sublime or excruciating, or both, depending on our environment.

Our difficulty accepting hierarchies of being that do not follow logic and our tendency to pick up on the emotions and sensations of other beings in our environment imbues Autistic people with a certain innate and intuitive animism. We empathize with beings whom our culture does not recognize as people: Whales, Cedars, stars, stones.

The older I got, the more that instinctual animism put me out of step with the world around me. And the grief and loneliness I felt deepened.

I knew that this world was in danger from people who did not understand that it was alive and who were willing to destroy it to get what they wanted. At nine, I could explain the dangers of nuclear winter and acid rain and was writing poetry about endangered species. At ten, I took a break from walking around the playground writing stories in my head to stand by the fence holding up homemade poster-board signs about Reagan's nuclear arms buildup for the passing cars to see. I did not understand how the people around me could be indifferent to the peril and the pain our culture's way of life was inflicting on the world.

The voices that made sense to me all came from other places and times and other worlds. My heart found strange solace in the melancholy beauty of the slow airs of my Irish ancestors and in the songs of Humpback Whales. In the fragments of understanding of Indigenous worldviews that came through in the books I could find in the library, I recognized that there were other ways of being human than the way the culture around me taught, and I found fainter traces of those same understandings in the English translations and modern interpretations of the folklore and myth of my Irish and Scottish and Norse ancestors. And in the poetry of William Butler Yeats, the novels of J. R. R. Tolkien, Susan Cooper, and Ursula LeGuin, and Carl Sagan's language of curiosity and wonder, I found the sense that I was not alone in sensing that other ways of being and seeing were possible and other worlds were close at hand.

And in the woods behind the house, walking through swampy soil that felt like it wanted to pull me down into the earth, those other worlds felt closer, and I could breathe more deeply.

The Maples, Oaks, and Birches were young, taking the place of trees that had been cleared in the centuries before to serve the needs of the people in the farm on the other side of the woods. But among them grew Skunk Cabbages born long before colonizers had come to the land.

Perhaps it was their presence that brought peace to my heavy young heart. Perhaps it was the memory held in the land itself—all the way down in the granite. Perhaps it was something else. All I know for certain is that the air felt different there to my asthmatic lungs that struggled so much with breathing in this world. It was not tinged with the same grief. And sometimes, from just beyond the edge of my field of vision, I would sense a shimmering presence that brought with it strange music that my heart could hear but my ears could not. There, I was not alone.

I stopped going into the woods sometime around when adolescence hit and began retreating entirely into my head. Asthma, a lack of coordination, and trouble navigating social situations made sports and gym class a nightmare for me, and I developed the sense that my body was broken, and that sensation and emotion were enemies. I never stopped believing that the world was alive, but I could not feel it fully when I did not feel like I, myself was fully alive.

As I came into adulthood, the fear I felt for the world remained and grew into outrage, but my sense of connection to the living world I wanted to save was fading into a mere abstraction. I spent my twenties and early thirties blockading weapons plants, documenting human rights atrocities, and reading, writing, and scheming about revolution. But no matter what I did, it never seemed commensurate with the level of suffering and destruction I was witnessing in the world, so I felt inadequate and kept trying to push myself further.

I was living a life in which I was deeply disconnected from my body—a lifetime of body shame overlapping with the remnants of a theology of martyrdom. I was struggling with asthma, depression, and insulin resistance that had me on the verge of diabetes. I was working more than full-time as a human rights activist for a small organization in Bangor, Maine, and viewed my body as a broken thing that mattered only as a vehicle for resisting the status quo, which seemed like the empire of modern myth. After a decade and a half of activism, I was feeling the futility of it all. So I threw myself into a war zone.

I went to Oaxaca, in southern Mexico, at a time when the city was occupied by military police who had come to crush an uprising. My heart was broken open by the strength of the people I met hiding in church basements, who had lived through horrors, and by the people I met in the mountains, who spoke of the land and the Corn as shaping their sense of who they were, which revealed exactly the empty place inside me from which the hunger for meaning arose.

Coming of age in this culture is a process of becoming "civilized"—a process of separating ourselves from the living world. My friend Stephen Buhner, who has now joined the ancestors, writes: "the word 'civilized' comes from the Latin *civilis,* meaning 'under law, orderly.' . . . *Civilis* itself comes from an older Latin word, *civis,* meaning 'someone who lives in a city, a citizen.'"[1]

It was Stephen who taught me that the first cities were defined by the walls built around them, separating them from the wilderness and the people who dwelled there, whose "Pagan" and "heathen" ways, ways "of the countryside," made them more loyal to the laws of nature than to the laws made by the people within the walls. This marked a catastrophic change in human history. My friend and teacher Cornelia Benavidez spoke about this with her teacher, the great American shaman Victor Anderson (whom we will meet more fully in the chapters to follow), and she communicated to me what Anderson had to say about the state of humankind.

> Victor inferred to me that humankind in modern times had to reframe
> the nature of nature that they had known for thousands of years in
> order to conquer not only it but all those in their way. Creating a new

kind of civilization. The reason or excuse for the carnage that took out entire tribes, villages, and kingdoms was the idea of order and control with the illusion of freedom through protection. This is not a bad idea if the system is reasonable and fair, but humankind went greedy and delusional resulting in what we are dealing with now on a worldwide level, which is an all-out assault on all life. He felt that this was the work of a filthy spirit that infected human kind with a great lie.

At first, the walls around the cities were necessary to mark the boundaries of the world subjected to that new order. Later, these evolved into walls along national borders—the Great Wall of China, Hadrian's Wall that separated Roman-occupied Britain from the untamable Scottish north, and the ditches and walls the British inheritors of that Roman order built, among them the palisade or pale (referring to the pales or stakes that constitute a fence) erected around Dublin. The Pale separated the part of Ireland around Dublin where the British had imposed their language, customs, and law from the Gaeilge-speaking places "beyond the Pale," where people still kept the old ways. Today, the walls are mainly abstract, barriers of access to the global financial system, largely maintained by that system, which has inherited the mantle of empire.

The walls exist within us too—in the form of ideas of acceptable thought and feeling that in time cause us to wall off perceptions that do not fit our worldview. As the brilliant and heretical Dr. Wilhelm Reich observed, these in turn become expressed in patterns of physical rigidity that constrict the flow of sensation.

The order imposed by this walling off of nature is illusory, of course. The living world has its own sense of order, one governed by a dynamic balance rather than a fixed rigidity, by curves and spirals rather than straight lines, and by infinite curiosity and creativity. What is rigid is brittle, prone to shatter when forces it seeks to resist or contain push strong enough and hard enough. And life, green and pulsing, always finds a way to break through—vines grow over walls, Dandelions grow up through the pavement, and human hearts break open.

In Oaxaca, I encountered people who, though having been subject to domination and oppression first by the Aztecs, then by the Spanish, and then by a Mexican state under the sway of U.S. geopolitical aims and the whims of global capital, had never allowed their hearts and spirits to be fully colonized and hence were never fully separated from the knowledge that the world was alive. In a Zapotec community in the hills, I met a man who held up a wooden carving of a wind spirit and said, "This is our inheritance—the gift of our ancestors is resistance." The sleeping spirit of my own inherent animism and my own inheritance of resistance stirred in response. When I returned to the United States, it awakened further.

The night that I came back I decided, for some reason, to go to a dinner party in Boston, something I would tend to view as nightmarish on the best of days, let alone when blown wide open. There was one person there whose presence felt different than anyone else's. When we finally spoke, she told me that she was an herbalist and began to speak of listening to the plants and of helping people regain connection with their own bodies. I was intrigued.

She called me a few weeks later, on New Year's Day, when I was sick with bronchitis. After we hung up, she called me back and said she had been listening to my breathing and knew the plant who could help me: "She has a bright yellow flower and a deep, resinous root and moves what we hold on to in our lungs. Her name is Elecampane."

When I took my first drops of Elecampane tincture that afternoon, I felt breath enter me deeply and experienced the unraveling of the story that my body was broken and could not be healed. I went walking in the snowy woods with my dog, breathing in the scent of Fir and Spruce and Pine, feeling my chest open wider and new life stir within me.

In the coming weeks, breath brought me more into my body, and I discovered how much I loved lifting heavy things. As weight lifting came into my life, my body started craving deeper nourishment, and, following my intuition, I started shifting how I ate, how I moved, and how I breathed.

Then, everything collapsed—an on-again, off-again romance that had broken open my heart finally came to an end at the same time that the funding ran out for my job. Believing that any path was better than the one I was on, I went walking in the Bangor (Maine) City Forest and prayed to get lost.

My eyes were drawn to the *Usnea* lichen that had fallen to the ground in the last rainstorm, its threads like the hair and beard of the wild Green Man of the forest. I followed the fallen *Usnea* until I found myself standing in a ring of Spruces I had never seen before. I closed my eyes and saw *Usnea*'s tendrils reaching into the cracked places in my heart.

I spent most of the following summer wandering through forest and field, listening deeply to the plants, and reading herb books at night.

When autumn came, I returned to the city, taking a job helping military families tell the stories of how the war in Iraq had devastated their lives. The wells of grief at the center of their hearts and mine seemed bottomless. I began to feel overwhelmed by despair again. So in the spring I went to the White Mountains of New Hampshire to listen to the forest.

By the third day of my vision quest, fasting alone in the forest, just above a stream flowing into the Pemigewasset River, it was all I could do to stumble to the edge of the ten-foot stone circle that marked the boundary of my world.

Just beyond that border, I saw a fallen Hemlock branch covered in lichen and, among the lichens, a patch of *Usnea* that seemed to glow with a pale light. To protect the trees that it grows on from infection, *Usnea* produces antibacterial and antifungal compounds that also serve as powerful medicine for humans and other animals.

From somewhere inside my chest, I heard the voice of the lichen speaking, telling me that the lichen would often grow in the places where the tree was wounded, that the wounds themselves called forth the medicine. A song began to rise inside me:

The wound is where the healing comes,
The wound is where the change begins!
Break on open and feel again,
Break on open and dream again,

Break on open and grow again,
Break on open and live again!

As I sang out loud, cycling through the chant again and again, questions and contradictions I had been struggling with began to resolve themselves.

Central was the conflict I felt between the political work I had dedicated my adult life to up to then and the healing work that I had been powerfully drawn to in recent years. More and more, it had been working to bring people together with plants that could support the healing of their bodies, minds, and spirits that had made me feel most alive. But strong voices inside me had been insisting that I had a responsibility to be part of political and cultural transformation.

That dichotomy fell away. I thought of the people who had come into my life and the pain they were living with—veterans, torture survivors, military families, refugees. And if—as *Usnea* was telling me—"the wound is where the change begins," then by coming to know the nature of those wounds, I would also come to know the wild, living medicines that could transform the culture that wounded them, healing hearts and healing worlds.

I left the world I had known behind, following the call of the plants. And as they worked through me, deeper and deeper layers of memory and knowing returned. The quest to awaken that memory further would take me to Ireland, where the living landscape of my own ancestors, and the remnants of ancient tradition that remained alive, would help me understand myself and the world more deeply.

This book is my best attempt to translate and share what I have learned from people and plants and gods and ancestors in the decade since I began to listen again to the voices of the living world. May it open the way for more people to begin to follow their own wild roads home.

The mountain is wreathed
by the smoke of burning forests
and across the ocean
pilots prepare

to set cities aflame.
But in this same world,
Bears crash through
thickets of huckleberries,
Salmon prepare for
their journey back
to the streams where
they were born,
and in autumn
Bears drag
the carcasses of Salmon
into the forest
where they
rot into the topsoil
and are reborn
as Cedar
and Trillium
and Wild Ginger.
Long ago
someone wrote
"Empires
rise and fall
but the mountains
and rivers
remain."

It is only because
we have forgotten
that we are dancing mountains
and flowing rivers
that we think
that the world
might end.

1
Living Medicine, Living Magic

Wherever there is soil and water, there are forests waiting to be reborn.

Along the Pripyat River in Ukraine, in the wake of the Chernobyl disaster, forests expanded to swallow up abandoned towns, and the Wolf and the Wild Boar have returned. For me that forest has come to symbolize the power of the wild to heal and transform even the most devastated landscapes when civilization gets out of the way.

That hope became a bit more fragile for me the day that I learned that forest was burning, set aflame by Russian artillery. As I read the news of those fires, I heard a Pileated Woodpecker drumming on a Spruce across the snowy yard.

Later that afternoon I was called to do a ritual for the healing of the Red Forest of Chernobyl. I found windblown Birch bark on the ground—a tree that connects me with the forests of Ukraine as well as my Irish and Swedish ancestral forests—which I gathered to use in place of an altar cloth. Then, I went to the old Spruce.

Where the Woodpecker had been drumming, the Spruce had poured out an amber resin—the color of the tears the Norse goddess Freyja, life of the land and teacher of the oldest magics, weeps. I lightly scraped the tree with the edge of a knife blade and gathered the golden tears in my hand.

At dusk, I spread the Birch bark out on my altar, lit a beeswax candle from a local beekeeper, heated a coal in my incense burner, and sprinkled the Spruce resin over the coal, calling forth a sweet cloud of smoke. I focused first on the flame of the candle and then on my heartbeat, calling up the memory of the Woodpecker's rhythm. I picked up my *bodhrán,* an Irish frame drum, and began playing the rhythm that memory stirred in my heart while holding the vision of the burning Red Forest being green again.

The Birch, the Spruce, and the Woodpecker had joined me in my prayer. And the first thing you must understand is that I am not speaking metaphorically.

My rite was not about my Will alone—it was the alignment of my Will with the living Will of the land. The Birch, the Spruce, the Woodpecker were part of an ecological community that holds the living knowledge of regeneration. My role was to bring the knowledge of distant fires to this place and ask for help.

The knowledge of those distant fires had changed the rhythms of my heartbeat and my breath and the pheromones my body was sending out as messenger molecules, taken in by trees that were inhaling my exhalations. The chemistry of the trees subtly changed in response, and so did the chemistry of the resins released by the drumming of the Woodpecker. And the bodies of the Woodpecker and I both responded to the aromatic molecules that wafted into the air from the resin, as did the other trees.

The biology of my own consciousness is a variation on the form of the mind of a forest. Trees and understory plants send down rhizomes, which intertwine with the mycelia that evolved to connect them, forming networks of filaments that carry chemical and electrical signals, allowing the land to experience itself simultaneously as myriad beings and one mind.

Human nervous systems, like all animal nervous systems, are networks of filaments, kin in form and function to the mycorrhizal networks that are the minds of forests and fields, contained within individual bodies. It was only very recently that we began to forget this, though there were always some cultures and communities and people who held on to this knowledge and allowed it to be the bedrock of their sense of being.

Something so recently forgotten can easily be remembered if we allow ourselves to open to it.

The trees of western Maine where I live are part of a forest with its own stories of resilience. Maine's forests were cut first to provide timber for the British navy a century after the forests my Irish ancestors loved faced the same fate, and then again and again to provide pulp for paper mills. Western Maine remained, in many ways, a colony of the logging and paper industries until the trade agreements of the early 2000s sent those industries south to Brazil. The forest has kept coming back. And while Wolves may not have returned here fully, though some believe they have begun to, I am serenaded at night by their descendants, Eastern Coyotes, a new species that evolved from the mating of Western Coyotes and Gray Wolves in Quebec.

As part of second- and third-growth forests, the trees around me know things I cannot know about how a forest regenerates after disaster. Having spent years cultivating a relationship with them, we are familiar with each other. So I call on them to help me shape my prayer, my spells, and my magic for a distant burning forest.

My relationship with them has changed what I understand magic to be. It has brought me to an understanding of magic that is wilder and older than most of what I have encountered in the modern Pagan world. And it is wilder, older magics that we need to remake worlds— and a living medicine that can help us remake ourselves.

In a time of fire, flood, and plague brought on in large part by centuries of human folly, it is wise to take another look at our ways of living, thinking, and relating to one another and to the living world. This requires us to look at how we understand and engage magic as well— because magic guided by the cultural logic that brought us to this place will not help us change course.

Whether or not they are aware of his influence on them, if asked to define magic, most modern Pagans and occultists would likely give an answer that echoes Aleister Crowley's famous dictum: "Magick is the art and science of creating change in conformity with Will." When we work with this definition, we can define medicine as a form of magic as well—the art and science of creating change within a human body in conformity with Will. (As my friend Dr. Mitchell Bebel Stargrove says, "Medicine and magick arise from the same gnosis—they are only separate if you make them so.") Crowley's definition of magick is a workable one, but it is one that begs an important question: Whose Will is being done?

Christianity famously answers this question with a phrase from the Lord's Prayer: "Thy will be done." St. Francis of Assisi prayed: "Make me an instrument of your peace." There is deep magic in this kind of surrender, and the god of Abraham is not the only entity to whom one can offer this devotion. An oracle offers this kind of devotion to a god or a goddess or a sacred spring. A soldier offers this same kind of devotion to the nation. This kind of deep surrender can allow fear and doubt to fall away, removing obstacles to the flow of power, making things that seemed impossible possible.

Yet, there are also dangers on this path. Christianity, Islam, and Vodun all warn that spirits are not always who they appear to be and that some will lie to gain surrender and cooperation from people. Even when gods and spirits are who they appear and claim to be, their interests may not be aligned with those of their servant—or of the family, community, nation, or world their servant is part of. Beings who demand absolute surrender—be they gods, spirits, people, or institutions—are often the last ones we should be trusting.

Another danger is that if we reduce ourselves to mere instruments of a greater Will, we are liable to treat other beings as instruments of that Will as well, whether they choose to be or not. Working in this framework, we are likely to see plants and animals and even other people as the property of the one we serve and justify treating them as objects to achieve the higher purpose we have dedicated ourselves to. In so doing, we lose touch with the sanctity of the rest of life and of the living world itself. As the great conservationist Aldo Leopold writes: "The last word in ignorance is the man who says of an animal or plant, 'What good is it?' If the land mechanism as a whole is good, then every part is good, whether we understand it or not."[1]

Going back at least as far as the Middle Ages, many occultists and ceremonial magicians have pushed back against Christianity's demand for surrender to the Will of the divine by elevating the individual Will and proclaiming, "My Will be done." In many ways this was the mindset that guided the Enlightenment for good and for ill. On the one hand, this brought a flourishing of individual freedoms, at least for the small class of people who were considered worthy and capable of exercising them. On the other hand, it became the basis by which people and nations justified taking what they needed to achieve their desires and defined land, water, forests, fields, plants, animals, and human labor as resources to be employed in realizing goals. In other words, it is tied to the very cultural logic that got us to this point. Because science and magic were a single discipline until the Enlightenment, our culture's approach to medicine is guided by this same logic. Our medicine seeks the power to change biological processes according to the desires of the doctor and the patient, desires that are shaped by the values of a culture that is increasingly separated from biological and spiritual reality. And at their deepest level, biological and spiritual realities are the same bedrock on which every other level of human reality rests. Whatever is not rooted in them is a tower built on a foundation of sand, just waiting to be brought down by a lightning strike or a strong wind—or a pandemic virus.

To be sure, the individual Will being enacted can be generous, merciful, and compassionate. Many magical traditions that work on building and focusing the individual Will also seek to ennoble that Will. For example, drawing on older traditions, Crowley's Thelema, a Western esoteric spiritual philosophy of the early 1900s, teaches that a true adept must achieve "congress with the Holy Guardian Angel"—that aspect of their being that is infinite and transcendent. In achieving this, however, we move beyond individualistic magic and personal Will into something resembling far older ways of engaging the world.

Animist magic, the original magic of people everywhere, seeks to partner with the living world. In the words of Caroline Casey, it is the "willingness to cooperate with everything"—a cooperation that requires honoring the dignity and sovereignty of all of life. Animist magic says, "Our Will be done." Done correctly it requires deep listening and communication and a willingness to understand that survival is a collective endeavor in which we are all dependent on one another.

Our individual Will does not vanish from the equation when we cooperate with everything. The Will of each being lending its voice to the prayer is heard. But as the rhythm of each voice entrains with the shared rhythm and its pitch and its movement come into complex harmony with other voices, what each Will sings into the song changes.

A growing number of physicists and biologists are gravitating toward animism, the understanding that the world itself is alive, and panpsychism, the understanding that there is intelligence in everything. Even those unwilling to use such language are increasingly acknowledging what chaos mathematics and systems theory began revealing half a century ago that our universe is full of complex, self-regulating systems that maintain balance and flow in nonlinear ways and learn and evolve in the process. Our ways of magic and medicine need to catch up with these understandings.

THE SEVEN COROLLARIES

There are certain corollaries that flow from the understanding that the world is alive that can serve as intellectual guideposts as we move forward. There are actually infinite corollaries that arise from this insight, but for now, I will focus on seven of them:

1. Our bodies are dynamic, complex living systems, and so is the body of our world.
2. Individual, community, cultural, and ecological health are inseparable.
3. There is an intelligence inherent in these interrelated complex living systems that will tend to maintain and, when necessary, protect and restore the integrity of the system.
4. Humans need connection with other humans and with other-than-human beings to maintain optimal health.
5. Plants and fungi are not inert materials for the production of medicine; they are living beings with their own intelligences. We seek to be in reciprocal relationship with the plants and fungi whose help we engage in healing.
6. Plants and fungi belong to themselves.
7. Beauty and wonder are ways we recognize the healthy flow of life.

Let's investigate these one by one.

1. Our bodies are dynamic, complex living systems, and so is the body of our world.

Separating mind from body and body from land, our culture has defined the land and waters as reservoirs of inert material and bodies as machines for transforming that material into wealth. Historian Silvia Federici writes:

> Capitalism was born from the separation of people from the land and its first task was to make work independent of the seasons and to lengthen the workday beyond the limits of our endurance. Generally, we stress the economic aspect of this process, the economic dependence capitalism has created on monetary relations, and its role in the formation of a wage proletariat. What we have not always seen is what the separation from the land and nature has meant for our body, which has been pauperized and stripped of the powers that pre-capitalist populations attributed to it.[2]

Outside the disciplines of mechanization visited on them, our bodies are capable of sensing subtle shifts in their experience of their internal ecologies—the intuitive dimensions of the pulse diagnosis come to mind—and in the world around us. Federici writes, "We know now, for instance, that the Polynesian populations used to travel the high seas at night with only their body as their compass, as they could tell from the vibrations of the waves the different ways to direct their boats to the shore"—which we can gloss as "reading the pulse of the ocean," just as an herbalist or acupuncturist can map the internal terrain of the body by feeling the way blood flows past particular points on the wrist.[3]

Bodies are constantly attuning to subtle flows within complex systems and to the ways in which everything shifts within and around them. Changes in complex systems can ultimately only be understood in terms of mapping the nature of such flows—whether through our senses, using our awareness of our own experience of embodiment as a technology of perception and investigation, or through the elaborate equations and algorithms of chaos mathematics and systems theory.

2. Individual, community, cultural, and ecological health are inseparable.

What is this thing I call a body, this community of cells and tissues and organs? It contains at least as many cells that we would call viral or bacterial or fungal as the cells we would call *Homo sapiens*. The elements that make it up are ancient—the hydrogen that combined with oxygen to form the water molecules that make up most of my body is older than the oldest stars. Yet the molecules and atoms contained in it have not been contained in it that long, comparatively; in fact, the mercury and dioxin stored in my superficial fascia when my body breathed them in and couldn't figure out how to neutralize or remove them in my childhood have been part of my body far longer than any of the molecules I can identify as part of my biochemistry. If anything, this body is another habitual way matter and energy have of arranging themselves. The water that flows through my body has flowed through other human and animal bodies, as well as through soil and roots and mycelia—and my health depends on the health of everything that water flows through. The soil is the fascia of Earth and what is contained within it will be held in my fascia as well. We are born of Earth's rain and oceans, its fire and lightning, and its minerals make up our bones. The space between our cells is like the space between stars, which is like the space between the electrons of an atom. This is not just poetic musing. It is—as Victor Anderson, the sage and Grand Master of the Feri tradition, would say—"the way things really are."

So, who is this persona who claims to be "me"? He is a product of the interaction of the consciousness that arises within my body with the actions and expressions of the other consciousnesses around me. If I spend most of my time in the forest, my persona will take on the characteristics of a forest. If I spend most of my time among other humans, my persona will take on characteristics of the community I participate in. The health of that persona, that psyche, is dependent on the health of the community that shapes it.

3. There is an intelligence inherent in these interrelated complex living systems that will tend to maintain and, when necessary, protect and restore the integrity of the system.

Most of contemporary Western biomedicine is guided by the belief that the body is a machine whose function is production and reproduction. Disease and injury are seen as the result of malfunctioning parts that will respond to manipulation, suppression, stimulation, replacement, or removal. Diagnosis is based on a taxonomy of symptoms, with little attention to their origin, and clusters of similar symptoms are treated identically.

Systems theory and complexity theory are revealing that model to be flawed and unscientific. Our bodies are not machines but self-organizing systems that adapt to change. The elements of those systems will always work in concert to ensure survival in the best ways that the information and resources available to it indicate. There is, in essence, no such thing as a maladaptive response; there are only responses based on faulty perception or wrong information, and often, unless there is significant organ damage, the only thing that can change the system's response is a change in the information the system has about the organism's experience of the world.

Simple things are easy for science to understand, explain, and predict. If you drop a ball, gravity will pull it toward the center of Earth, causing it to fall. Other factors also come into play—the speed and direction of the wind, the height and angle from which you drop the ball—but they are easy to factor in. You can come up with an equation that will reliably predict when and where the ball will hit the ground. When we begin to look at more complex phenomena, like weather, simple models don't work as well to explain what is happening. This is why a weather forecast is likely to be less accurate than predictions about dropped balls.

Edward Lorenz, who worked on early computer models of the atmosphere, discovered that exceedingly small changes in one part of a system could create big changes in another part of the system. He would become famous for making the analogy that a butterfly flapping its wings in one part of the world could create—or prevent—a tornado in a distant part of the planet. Describing such events is one thing, predicting them is another, made complicated by the fact that every element of a large, complex system has its own complex and ever-changing behaviors and is made up of nesting systems with their own complexity. The way the temperature and currents of lake water change the weather is a smaller version of the ways in which the temperature and currents of an ocean affect it, and both are microcosms in liquid form of the great ocean of air that is Earth's atmosphere.

If we see the mathematics and physics of our dominant culture as having their roots in the rationalist natural philosophy of classical Athens, then we can say that it took Western science millennia to begin to grasp these complexities. It took two millennia for the innate knowledge the ancient Greeks accessed through their use of an ergot fungus to reappear through the mind-altering substance LSD. Athenian philosophers were initiated into the mysteries of Eleusis with the help of *kykeon,* a brew made from *Claviceps purpurea.* When their intellectual descendants rediscovered that fungal medicine through a semisynthetic form of one of its key alkaloids, lysergic acid diethylmide-25, the fractal realities mathematics describes became clear to Western minds.

Indigenous science, working with embodied intuition and with knowledge that arises from direct connection to the wind and rain and snow and sun and the living world around us, has always had more nuanced and accurate ways of predicting and describing changes in weather than conventional meteorology has. The same is true of our bodies. We can see the conditions within our body as our internal weather, and changes in our body, like changes in the planet's weather, can never be entirely understood or described in linear ways. The longer a condition endures, the truer this becomes.

Let's look at hypertension, for example. A person afflicted with high blood pressure consults a physican and an herbalist. The patient perceives the world as in some way unsafe, and so the body has elevated its blood pressure to be ready to respond to those threats. To lower blood pressure, the physician gives hydrochlorothiazide, and the herbalist gives Dandelion (*Taraxacum officinale*), both of which increase urination, reducing the volume of fluids in the body and thus reducing blood pressure. That works for a while, but the person still perceives the world as unsafe, and so in response to the drug and the herb, the body increases angiotensin to increase arterial tension. The physician then gives an angiotensin-converting enzyme (ACE) inhibitor, and the herbalist responds with Reishi (*Ganoderma lucidum*). Again, because the perception of threat remains, the body makes an end-run around the process by increasing levels of norepinephrine. So the physician gives a beta-blocker to shut down the beta receptor sites for norepinephrine, and the herbalist gives an adaptogen. Whatever response the practitioners bring, the body keeps finding new ways to elevate the blood pressure, because elevating blood pressure is an adaptive response to living under constant threat.

Except that when the herbalist gives Dandelion or Reishi, another intelligence becomes involved in the process. This happens whether the clinician or the patient is aware that it is happening, though it happens more effectively when the conscious Wills of all involved are in cooperation. Dandelion, with its resilience and its root's knowledge of water, encourages a fluid release not just of the excess moisture in the body, but also of the water-soluble biological metabolites created by past experiences that are driving the fear. Reishi, which has digested the memories held in the wood of trees, goes deeper still, metabolizing memories held within the body and sending its mycelial intelligence into the spaces left behind, bringing awareness of connection. And rewoven into the intelligence of the living world, the patient can begin to release the fear and pain that made the world feel dangerous in ways that made him or her tense against its threats and elevate blood pressure. Changing the information coming into the system changes the dynamic flow.

From the *qi* of Chinese medicine and the *prana* of Ayurveda to the vital force of nineteenth-century physiomedicalist herbalism, people around the world and throughout history have spoken of a force that moves coherently through the body, giving life to its organs and tissues. When it flows properly, we experience health. When its flow is blocked or reduced—or when it burns too hot and fast—we experience disease.

Working in the first half of the twentieth century, psychologist and biophysicist Wilhelm Reich observed this moving, pulsing energy at work in human bodies and in the simplest life-forms. He called it orgone and noted that its motion—its expression—was guided by sensory information.

Living nature, in contrast to the nonliving, responds to stimuli with "movement" or "motion" = "emotion." It necessarily follows, from the functional identity of emotion and plasmatic movement, that even the most primitive flakes of protoplasm have sensations. The sensations can be understood directly from the responses to stimuli. These responses of plasmatic flakes do not differ in any way from those of highly developed organisms. There are no lines to be drawn here.[4]

Today, we know that slime molds can learn and alter their behavior according to sensory stimuli and that complex signals sent between plants along mycelial networks result in plants receiving new information and altering their chemistry. We, too, respond to sensory information. Part of that sensory information is the set of electromagnetic fluctuations detected by neurons in the heart that the amygdala and the right frontal cortex of the brain interpret as emotion (for more on this, see Stephen Buhner's *The Secret Teachings of Plants*).

Reich noted that tension in the muscles and fascia blocks the flow of orgone through the body, resulting in changed behaviors at the level of tissue, organ, organism, and consciousness. Rigidity restricts motion. Motion defines life. The invitation back into motion comes through eliciting changes in sensation.

He observed particles of orgone that he called bions. Most of Reich's scientific colleagues rejected his theories and findings on ideological grounds, without investigating them themselves. However, contemporary biophysicists' description of biophotons, weak photons emitted from the DNA at the nucleus of a cell, bear an uncanny similarity to Reich's description of the bions he saw in his microscope in both living and decaying tissues.

Our life and our bodies are not apart from the rest of the living universe. Reich observed and worked with orgone in our atmosphere, and he perceived it as animating stars and galaxies. To put it in more expressly animist terms than Reich himself used, the forms of stars and clouds and people and animals and plants are particular arrangements that matter and energy take on for the purpose of experiencing the universe. Animist herbalism seeks to remove obstacles to the flow of life through us and to nourish that flow until the matter and energy contained within us yearn for dissolution.

Every response of a cell, a tissue, an organ, an organism, or a community—be it a physiological or behavioral response—is the system's best attempt to meet its needs with the resources and information available. The task of the healer is to understand what the system is responding to and why it is responding the way it is responding. If we seek to change the response, we need to change the information driving the response or give the system another way to accomplish what it needs to accomplish. That change in information needs to be a change in sensory information.

4. Humans need connection with other humans and with other-than-human beings to maintain optimal health.

Our ancestors evolved in a world that they experienced as alive and connected to them, speaking to them in many ways. Their bodies were attuned to the rhythms of wind and water, the sound of the air moving beneath an Eagle's wing, the exhalations of Cedar and Honeysuckle and Datura, the scents in the air, and the pheromones of desire in each other's heartbeats.

Our biology is much the same as theirs, but our lives today are full of threats and assaults and noise that we cannot make sense of. When we experience things that overwhelm our senses, and when we experience situations in which we cannot imagine a positive or even acceptable outcome, we become disconnected from ourselves. Our cognitive capacities decline and then shut down, our sense of what is happening within our bodies and in the world around us becomes narrowed to our perception of the most immediate threat in our world, and we prepare to deal with that threat, alone, by fighting, fleeing, or freezing. Our immune responses become dysregulated, as the body releases inflammatory compounds intended to deal with any injury that might result from the threat. Our digestion goes offline. Our heart beats too quickly or too slowly and gets stuck in that response. Our blood sugar and blood pressure spike.

We come back into regulation by coming back into connection with our own bodies and our own web of relations. Most forms of psychotherapy seek to bring us into regulation by helping us come into healthy relationships with other humans. But human relationships are not the only relationships that can be therapeutic.

Connecting with plants, animals, and fungi can help to draw us back into embodied presence—especially if our history of human interactions is fraught with pain, fear, and struggle. We have an immediate, visceral set of responses to the presence of plants. When we breathe in their scents, our smooth muscles relax, we become more sensitive to hormonal signals inside and around us, and our nervous systems move into a state of coherence that recalibrates the function of our internal organs. As Guido Masé writes, "aromatics bring us into focused, flowing balance and help us function more efficiently."[5] We seek the shade of trees in summer, and the kiss of blades of grass glazed with dew.

They are our wild kin. They bring us profound medicine. And that kinship is part of the medicine.

5. Plants and fungi are not inert materials for the production of medicine; they are living beings with their own intelligences. We seek to be in reciprocal relationship with the plants and fungi whose help we engage in healing.

This reciprocal relationship includes supporting the health of wild populations of plants and fungi that we call upon for our medicine and magic and the health of their ecosystems. I tend to work with very small doses of herbal and fungal medicines—one to five drops of a tincture at a time, just enough to give the body new sensory information so that fewer plants and fungi need to give their bodies and their lives to transforming human experiences. Matthew Wood introduced a generation of herbalists to the practice of drop dosing—a practice he learned from the writings of the Eclectic physicians of the nineteenth century.

Herbal medicines given at minute doses can instigate profound shifts in our sensory and emotional experiences. Indeed, to some extent, small "energetic" or "spirit" doses of herbs are most effective at instigating such shifts, because, with a few exceptions, they tend to be below the threshold of pharmacological activity and hence do not bring direct stimulation or sedation of particular organ functions. If you have felt a drop of Rose tincture soften and open your heart—and perhaps bring on tears—then you have experienced this phenomenon.

Our nervous and endocrine systems evolved responding to minute phytochemical inputs in the air our ancestors breathed, the water they drank, the brush of leaf and petal against their skin. We can replicate those exposures with drop doses of tinctures (as well as with having people spend time in the presence of aromatic herbs). The very fact that we innately recognize that these are the chemical and electromagnetic touch of other life forms, wild kindred, increases the salience of those experiences. When we cannot bring people to the forest, we can bring something of the forest to them. When I can send someone to the forest or the field, sometimes I do not take herbs internally at all; instead, I may send them to visit a plant.

Out of respect for the plants and fungi that are involved in my healing work, my therapeutic goals always have an ecological dimension. I seek to help people regain their ability to perceive and act in accordance with their connection to and interdependence with the other members of the human and other-than-human communities they belong to by bringing them into states of openhearted embodied presence. I do not seek to make it easier for people to continue to participate in an ecocidal culture. I especially do not disrespect the lives of the plants and fungi whose bodies we use as medicine by using them to enable the continuation of ways of being and thinking and seeing and feeling and unfeeling that threaten the well-being of their kin.

6. Plants and fungi belong to themselves.

While traditional relationships between plants and fungi and the Indigenous cultures that arose alongside them need to be honored as part of the ecology of a place, plant and fungal knowledge is a continuing revelation arising from all authentic and sincere relationships with the plants and fungi themselves. Honoring those traditional relationships is akin to honoring a person's relationships with the other people in his or her life. It is important to be respectful, but also important to make your own relationship on your own shared terms.

For many years, I lived in a bioregion where Devil's Club grows. Coast Salish peoples have long engaged the plant in protection magic, but though their ritual, medical science, and technology inform my understanding of the plant, I do not engage it using their cultural practices. I came to know Devil's Club on its own terms and visited it regularly, bringing offerings and prayers and harvesting it according to instructions the plant itself gave me.

I can tell you that Devil's Club grows where the forest has been disrupted by a clear-cut, a landslide, or a flood. It protects rich soils and the wildflowers that grow in them because its spiky stalks prevent big creatures from blundering over them, and its great leaves shade the ground. I can tell you that it is so hard to remove by hand that it stopped the northward expansion of the railroads in British Columbia. I can tell you its green buds tipped with purple pulse with life in spring.

But though I tell you these things about the plant, you still do not know Devil's Club. Devil's Club will not be ready to join you in your work until you have made your own relationship with it. And when you do, your magic and medicine will not resemble mine—except in the ways that they are both touched by Devil's Club's unmistakable presence.

7. Beauty and wonder are ways we recognize the healthy flow of life.

Our innate aesthetic sense is rooted in our emotional response to the sensory signals flowing into us from the outside world. This gets complicated and distorted by the aesthetic ideals our conscious mind absorbs from our cultures, which are shaped by the culture's ideology. When we train ourselves to shift our aesthetic response away from the learned judgments of our talking, thinking minds and toward the responses of our hearts and our bodies as a whole, we begin to perceive beauty wherever there is healthy flow. The meaning we make creates context for memories and experiences, new and old. The structure of our brain shifts accordingly.

Our aesthetic sense is also deeply connected with our capacity to recognize patterns, especially those patterns that represent the relation-

ship between forms and functions. The Irish god Manannán Mac Lir
sees the sea as a field of wildflowers. The Zen poet Dōgen saw mountains as slowly moving rivers of stone and rivers as swiftly moving
mountains of water. I see all these things and more. In my worldview,
it is not mere whimsy to equate a river and a galaxy. Both are alive and
flowing. And so are you. And so am I. And so are we.

The architect Louis Sullivan had the famous insight that form follows function. We see this in the way that the branching networks of
information exchange between plants and fungi—the intertwining
of plant rhizomes and fungal mycelia—resemble the structure of the
human nervous system. The same pattern repeats when we map the
distribution of galaxies in the known universe and superimpose their
forms and placement onto their lines of connection—a fact with profound cosmological implications that suggest that not only is the planet
alive and conscious but the universe itself may be as well. The ability to recognize these patterns is mediated in large part by the indole
alkaloids—molecules like serotonin and dimethyltryptamine and mela-
tonin and their cousins psilocybin and lysergic acid diethylamide, which
our fungal and plant and bacterial ancestors evolved to facilitate information flows through complex webs of consciousness.

Herbalists have long looked at the physical form of plants' bodies
for clues to how they will work with human bodies, a principle known
as the doctrine of signatures. There is a crude and easily ridiculed version of this principle that tends to be reduced to memorized sets of correspondences divorced from embodied experience. A more subtle and
nuanced approach to recognizing signatures comes from meditation on
the form of a plant. The heterodox Christian philosophers Paracelsus
and Jakob Boehme—whose writings defined Western understandings of
the doctrine in the sixteenth and seventeenth centuries—both believed,
as Matthew Wood writes, that "the whole natural world corresponds
to the archetypal world, which gives it form and meaning."[6] In other
words, the physical form of any life-form is a reflection not only of its
function but also of its essential nature, the qualities that make an Oak

an Oak, a Dolphin a Dolphin, and a person a person. As living beings, we have the innate capacity to understand this language of form at an intuitive level. Wood's own work provides beautiful examples of how a contemporary herbalist can use the doctrine of signatures to discover overlooked and novel dimensions of a plant's medicine.

This is true at the molecular level as well: molecules with similar structures tend to have similar functions and tend to show up in parts of organisms that have similar forms and functions. For example, the human body uses the neurotransmitter serotonin to stimulate the growth of new neural connections. Plants use either serotonin or auxin, a rooting hormone with a serotonin-like molecular structure, to stimulate rhizomic growth. The *Psilocybe cubensis* mushroom uses psilocybin and psilocin to stimulate mycelial growth. These compounds also stimulate root growth in the grasses *Psilocybe cubensis* grows with symbiotically, and they stimulate the formation of new synaptic connections in human brains. Stephen Buhner goes into this eloquently and at great length in his book *Plant Intelligence and the Imaginal Realm*, and I will touch on this biology again later in this book.

Our bodies intuitively recognize this chemistry through the ways they respond to the scents and tastes of plants and the somatic shifts their constituents create in the body. Understandings of plant medicines rooted in direct, embodied experience tend to outpace those based on pharmacology by decades or even centuries. Aesthetics are also central to good herbal formulation. A proper herbal formula will feel like a single herb to the body and will engage the senses fully. My medicine is also a bardic medicine that begins to break down the distinction between the literal and the metaphorical. What we call the literal is an attempt to impose a single set of colonial metaphors on the world. What we call the metaphorical can be a potent tool for changing the meaning of information, sensations, and experiences by giving them new context.

Together, these seven principles underlie and give rise to a system of healing that honors the intelligence and life of our bodies and of the living world from which they arise. At its core, this approach to healing is about creating the conditions that allow for healthy flow. We can shift that flow through sensory impulses that stimulate the body to respond differently. Those sensory experiences create new synaptic connections when they are novel and reinforce existing ones when they are repeated. We, quite literally, come to our senses.

Hot, spicy things stimulate the flow of blood and sensation. The aromatic scents of plants invite the opening of the senses. Bitter tastes stimulate the part of the nervous system in the gut, bringing us grounding. The acrid taste—the sensation of burning at the back of the throat—induces muscular relaxation, as do profoundly bitter tastes. The sweet taste brings a sense of nourishment.

Also, color has its purpose and meaning in plants and is taken into account consciously and subconsciously. From the aurora borealis to our electric body, does it not make sense that color gives us clues to our healing just as it gives clues to our condition? We intuitively recognize that when tissues are redder than usual, they are experiencing inflammation. We don't need the intellectual understanding of the fact that the redness arises from an increased flow of oxygenated blood into those tissues, though such an understanding does give context for the meaning we derive from seeing tissues turn red. Color is an important part of the signatures of plants as well: the deep red of Hawthorn berries, for example, evokes thoughts of blood and of heat, and Hawthorn is a profound medicine for inflammation in our blood vessels.

All of these sensations change what it feels like to inhabit a body in a particular moment, which changes the way the body responds. When we feel safe and free, movement, sensation, and blood flow freely through the body, promoting healthy organ function and the growth and repair of tissues. When we feel afraid or overwhelmed, that flow is blocked. When we feel depressed, that flow is diminished.

The most salient experiences we have create the strongest memories. The neural connections created by those memories are strengthened each time we repeat or remember those experiences. Those memories, in turn, shape the way we perceive new sensations and experiences. They shape what we notice, what we register as significant, and what meaning and context, both conscious and subconscious, that we give to events in our inner and outer worlds.

This is not to say that disease is the result of negative thinking. What I am speaking about is not a question of thought or belief, but rather a question of what it feels like to be you in the world in this moment and the way your body interprets and acts on that feeling.

THE THREEFOLD SELF

For me, the distinction works best when I think about the model of the threefold self that I learned to work with during my training as a priest of the Feri tradition, a shamanic tradition that found its modern expression on the West Coast of North America in the second half of the twentieth century, through the teachings of Victor Anderson.

From an early age, Victor was mostly blind and profoundly psychically gifted. Past life memories and spirit visitations began coming to him as a child. Native, Mexican, and African healers and shamans in the communities, or passing through where he grew up, in New Mexico and Oregon, recognized his gifts and worked to heal and train him, much to his mother's consternation. As a young adult in the 1930s, he found a coven of witches in Ashland, Oregon, who invited him to join them. Several years later he met and married Cora Ann Cremeans, who had grown up in Alabama, having her own spirit encounters and learning bits of Irish and Scots-Irish folk magic from her grandfather, who was called a druid. Others in Alabama, from kind Christians who did not frown on folkways to mysterious people and her own paranormal experiences and dreams, helped her to recognize Victor as her soulmate. Their marriage and their shared practice, along with Victor's wide reading and profound intuition, shaped the insights, orientation, cosmology, ethics, and practices that would become known as the Feri tradition. One of their early initiates, Gwydion Pendderwen, whom Victor considered a spiritual son, brought more Irish and Welsh elements into the tradition as it developed. (For a sense of that approach and of who Victor was, see *Victor Anderson: An American Shaman* by Cornelia Benavidez.)

Victor noted that many societies throughout history have worked with threefold models of the self. He spoke most frequently of Hawai'ian, Yoruban, and kabbalistic expressions of this concept, but he also recognized its presence in the three cauldrons, or three fires, of the Irish tradition and in the Christian Trinity. Others have pointed to analogues in Vedic and Taoist systems. For simplicity's sake, I will refer to these three selves by descriptive English names used by some of us in the tradition: the Human Self, the Animal Self, and the God Self. Matthew Wood works with a similar system derived from Hawai'ian tradition as interpreted by the missionary and scholar Max Freedom Long, who partially saw it through the lens of a Judeo-Christian worldview.

What we call the Human Self is the part of us that operates in the realm of words, symbols, ideas, beliefs, categories, and abstractions. We can roughly understand it as having its seat in the left frontal cortex of the brain. It is what gives form to art, what drives science, what inspires technology. It is also the only aspect of the self that the dominant culture validates and gives voice to. Disconnected from the rest of our being, it tends to become rigid and tyrannical. As Wilhelm Reich wrote, "The more the thought process is removed from reality, the more intolerance and cruelty are needed to guarantee its continued existence."[7]

The Animal Self is the part of ourselves that experiences sensation and emotion. We can roughly understand it as having its seat in the neurological nexus that involves the nerves of the genitals; the enteric nervous system, or "gut brain," which not only regulates digestion but also senses the electromagnetic and kinetic information moving through the fascia of the rest of the body; the neurons of the heart, which sense electromagnetic change in our inner and outer worlds; the amygdala, which filters and processes those signals along with the information coming in from the hormonal content of the blood; and the right frontal cortex of the brain, which assigns meaning to all of this. The Animal Self knows things not by what they are called or how they are categorized, but by how they feel. It thrives on pleasure and loving connection. It holds the memory of trauma and helps us avoid repeating devastating events by making us react strongly to the sensations associated with them. The stories the Human Self tells about the world evoke particular emotional responses from the Animal Self. It often experiences the judgments of the Human Self as instilling guilt, shame, and fear, which it also tries to avoid. Its experience of the world is the felt sense that governs our body's physiological responses to what is happening within and around us. Disconnected from the rest of our being, it tends to pursue pleasure and avoid pain without contextualizing them in a broader framework of experience. In connection with the world, it is capable of feeling things the Human Self cannot yet imagine and conveying to it new senses of possibility.

The God Self is the part of us that understands our own infinity. This is more than a theological concept. The more we understand our own bodies, the more we understand that we are microcosms that contain countless species acting symbiotically to support the continuation of one experience, one consciousness. In turn, these countless species are part of a larger macrocosm of human, ecological, and, ultimately, cosmic connection. There is no fixed boundary to who we are, where we begin and end. The matter and energy contained within our bodies is recycled and exchanged with the world around us over and over again and exists in dynamic relationship with the rest of the matter and the energy in the universe. This is a concept the Human Self cannot fully comprehend, but in moments of profound opening, our Animal Self experiences that reality viscerally. The sensations and emotions of the Animal Self are received by the God Self as a kind of somatic prayer.

Intervening at the level of belief and thought is intervening at the level of the Human Self and will often have little effect on the felt sense of being alive, except to the extent that shifting its judgments can sometimes partially shift emotional responses to a part of someone's inner or outer world. We change the experience of the Animal Self by changing what it feels, shifting its reality by engaging the senses, creating somatic shifts that, in turn, present the Animal Self with a new reality to map and imagine and that open the way to connection with the world beyond us, including our own infinity. Such shifts are not bounded by cultural limitations, except in so far as we experience the judgment of the Human Self. The Human Self responds to those new experiences in one of two ways: it either changes its structure of beliefs, and hence our brain structure, to accommodate the new experiences, or it changes the memory and meaning of those experiences to fit into its existing belief structures. So we can gain its cooperation by giving it a story that makes sense within the framework of its own worldview that gives context to the changes that are about to ensue. It is for this reason that I will speak in the pages to come in mythic, historical, and scientific terms, in ways that seek to invite the Human Self back into community with the rest of life.

LISTENING TO TREES

To seek change on the level required to heal ourselves and the world, we need to bring our own Wills into cooperation with other-than-human Wills. This requires approaching our wild kin with openness, curiosity, and respect.

If you want to generate rain, the best magic you can work is to grow a forest. Years ago in Nicaragua, a group of farmers told me the story of how they did just this. These farmers had all grown up hearing stories of the monsoons their parents and grandparents depended on to keep their farms fertile. In those days, their community had been surrounded by forests. Under the Somoza dictatorship, the trees were cut down and sold off. When the forest was gone, the monsoons stopped coming. After the revolution that overthrew the Somoza regime in 1979, the community came together and began to plant trees. Trees do not make a forest by themselves, but underground seeds and spores and roots and mycelia remained and responded to the return of the trees, and as the trees grew, the forest returned. It took decades, but by 2005 the monsoons had returned, and their crops were flourishing.

If you want rain but do not have time to grow a forest, you can try speaking with the wind and the clouds themselves, just as all of our ancestors once did (and some people still do.) But these forces are immense and often impersonal, and if you have lived all your life not knowing that the world is alive and not engaging the world around you, you are unlikely to be able to convince them to listen to you. Better to start with something more like you—for example, a tree. But before a tree will listen to you, you need to spend time listening to a tree. Listening to trees is a very old way to learn magic.

The modern word *druid* (and the Irish word *draoi*, which means "magician or sorcerer") is derived from two Proto-Indo-European words that go back to the Neolithic: *deru*, which means "tree" (preserved in the modern Irish and Welsh names for the Oak—*dair* and *derr*), and *wyd*, which means "to see or to know." Trees are memory keepers, beings whose bodies hold the record of all that has come to pass in a particular place for centuries—whether they lived through those events themselves or carry the inherited memory from their predecessors and from the soil and the water. In old understandings, to work magic requires learning to see the world as a tree does. The trees themselves are teachers.

◊ Deepening Kinship with Trees ◊

Many of the old ways of apprenticing to a tree are lost, but I have adapted and expanded a simple practice from the work of Stephen Buhner and Julie McIntyre and have found it to be a profound way of beginning to learn from trees.

First, find a tree in the landscape you inhabit that calls to you.

Bring your attention to the beating of your own heart. As you feel your heartbeat, think of how your heart has beat for you in every moment of your life, through wild joy and deep sorrow, without your ever needing to ask it to. Let gratitude arise like a wild spring from the center of your heart and fill it. Bless your blood so that it flows throughout your body and

comes out with your breath, blessing the world. Let that gratitude come back in with your next in-breath.

With your next inhalation, feel that gratitude coming in
with your breath, flowing toward your heart. Let your attention
expand from your heart down to your root. Let your awareness move from your own root down into the soil and grow
tendrils that intertwine with the roots and rhizomes of the tree
you seek to connect with.

Now allow yourself to feel the presence of the tree. Allow
images, sensations, scents, memories, fragments of song to
arise. Be present with them without yet attempting to assign
them meaning. Don't worry if there are no words—as long as
you have allowed yourself to feel the presence of the tree, on
its own terms, you have done what is required.

When you are ready, thank the tree, and then draw your
awareness back up through your root to your heart. Pay attention again to your own heartbeat and thank your heart. Run
your hands over your own body, with a firm touch, letting
yourself feel your boundaries and your solidity. Take some time
to record and reflect on what you experienced and learned.

Make a schedule for visiting the tree, and do not deviate
from it. Each time you visit the tree, bring a gift that is deeply
meaningful to you. Most often, I bring whiskey or honey. I
don't know for certain what the tree makes of the honey or
the whiskey themselves, but I know that bringing them changes
the way I show up, and that trees respond to that difference.

Over time, you will develop a felt sense of the presence of
that tree. Learn to recognize its particular form, textures, and
scents and the way your breath and your heartbeat respond
to its presence. Practice calling up the memory of these sensations until you can conjure up a sense of the tree's presence
wherever you are, just as you would conjure the felt sense of
the remembered presence of a person you love.

Begin to recognize what the tree itself needs and wants and desires. Let these be questions in your heart each time you visit. When the tree begins to answer in ways that do not align with your assumptions of what it needs, you have learned to listen well. Having learned to listen, begin performing acts of care and generosity for your sylvan companion.

You will likely notice, too, that, just as you take on the postures and mannerisms and turns of phrase of people you spend time with, the nature of your own presence will change the more you spend time with the tree. Cherish these changes and cultivate the ways of being the tree is teaching you.

This process can last a lifetime, but there will come a time when you have a clear sense that you and the tree have become deep allies. You may come to know it in a dream, or you may just notice in the waking world that your relationship with this tree has become more intimate. When this has taken place, besides listening to the tree's deep desires, you can begin bringing your own heart's questions and concerns to the tree. Pay attention in the days that follow to dreams, synchronicities, memories, and new information that make themselves known.

Now that you have reached the beginning place, you are ready to begin weaving magic together with this tree. Come to your tree only with prayers for transformation that are aligned with the nature and interest of the tree and its kin. Take only what the tree offers freely. Stand with it, holding in your body the sense of the change in the world you desire. Allow the tree to change the shape of that desire. And together, breathe it to the wind.

This is the heart of animist plant magic. All else is a variation on this simple beginning.

From this beginning place, we set down roots that entwine with the roots of that tree. Like all roots, those roots will seek water. Let us follow them downward now.

The water
that flows
within you

is the river
of stars,

flowing
from the well
which whispers
the secret names
of all things,

which arise
within you
anew,

becoming
the clouds
and the thunder

that rain down
worlds,
to bring the lightning
that sets life
in dancing motion.

2
The Otherworld Well

For as long as I can remember, my Da has brought holy water from the shrine of Our Lady of Knock when visiting people in the hospital—a quiet, humble ministry that has its recent origins in rituals of the Irish Catholic diaspora, but deep roots in far older traditions of our people.

Knock is a village in County Mayo in the west of Ireland, where, on a late August evening in 1879, people coming home from gathering hay or harvesting turf in preparation for the coming winter witnessed the appearance of Mary, dressed in white robes and holding a golden Rose and attended by Saint Joseph and Saint John the Evangelist.

This was a generation after An Gorta Mór, the Great Hunger, brought on by the British demand that Ireland keep exporting food to its colonial masters while the potatoes the Irish people had depended on for sustenance were destroyed by late blight. Potatoes had been the principal food for the Irish since the destruction of older food sources during the scorched-earth campaign of the British commander Oliver Cromwell two centuries earlier. It had been, in many ways, a second wave of the same genocide the people's great-grandparents had survived or perished in. During the time of hunger, people wandered from town to town searching for food, many collapsing in the streets. They were buried in mass graves that held thousands. Others, huddled in cottages, died of diseases that spread rapidly through a traumatized and malnourished population. People called out to Mary, to Jesus, to Saint Brighid, and, in some places, to older spirits as well for mercy and aid. To those who survived and to their children who grew up under occupation from the same forces that had allowed so many to die preventable deaths, Mary's apparition at Knock was an affirmation that their prayers had not gone unheard.

Our Lady of Knock played an important role in my childhood religion: among the descendants of Daniel O'Donoghue and Nora O'Meara in the heavily Irish Catholic parishes north of Boston, there was never a funeral or a memorial service where we did not sing her hymn. The hymn bore a promise that "the Lamb will conquer, and the woman who holds up the sun will shine her light on everyone."[1]

That image of the woman holding up the sun conjures the image of figures far older than the mother of Jesus: the first is Áine, solar goddess of abundance, venerated at Midsummer, ancestor and one of the sovereignty goddesses of the Eóghanact tribe of which the O'Donoghues are a branch. (Every Irish tribe traces its descent back to the husband or son of a goddess of the land—a goddess to whom kings and chieftains are ritually wed.) The second is Brighid of the bright flame, a goddess whose name and mantle would be taken on by a Catholic saint said to be the midwife of Christ. Saint Brighid is second only to Mary and Jesus in her level of veneration among the Irish and the Irish diaspora, and anyone who has spent time in an Irish Catholic house on either side of the Atlantic will know that Mary is venerated to an equal or greater degree than her son.

The name of the site of that Marian apparition, Knock, is an anglicization of the Irish Gaeilge word *cnoc,* which means "hill" or "mound." An older near synonym for cnoc is *sidhe*—a word that refers both to the burial mounds of Ireland's pre-Gaelic Neolithic tribes and to the beings the old gods, from whom the modern Irish people trace the oldest indigenous side of their roots, became when they vanished from the world to escape the onslaught of a civilization whose ways were too brutal for them. We can think of the font of holy water at the shrine of Our Lady of Knock as taking the older place of the well near the burial ground as a place for calling on healing from the source of all life—a connection I only really understood once I was in Ireland.

In Liscannor, just south of the Cliffs of Moher on the rocky coast of County Clare, there is a well fed by a cold, wild spring, where Brighid was honored once as a goddess and now as a saint. The well is at the foot of a mound where new and old graves stand above the ancient tombs of chieftains and kings, buried close to the waters that could carry them into the arms of their wild lover, the land itself to which they were ritually wed at their coronations. A short way up the hill is a clootie tree—a tree where people tie strips of cloth as they pray for the health of their families and the fertility of their land.

In the first days of September, in 2017, I found myself standing by the tree, looking down toward the well, praying for the healing of the forests I had just learned were burning in the Columbia River Gorge where I then made my home. Hearing a voice echo within me saying, "A big prayer requires a big offering," I hung one of my most prized possessions from a branch—the tip of a Deer antler on a rawhide string given to me by someone I loved when I first came to the gorge.

I went down to the well itself, contained now by stone walls lined with photos of the sick and the dead, Brighid's crosses woven with reeds, and candles burning in small grottoes, drank deeply of the cold, cold water, light brown with the tannins of the peat it had filtered through.

There was a steady stream of people coming, bearing photographs and rosaries, even on a weekday morning. After making their prayers, many would gaze into the water. Tradition says that if you see an image of a Salmon in the play of light and shadows on the water, the person you are praying for will be healed: echoes of a still older way of seeing the world.

There is no surviving evidence of an Irish creation story—perhaps the birth and origin of the world is not as universal a fascination as our contemporary culture assumes. But the origin of springs and rivers is another question—though as much a geographical question as a temporal one, but no less definitive of a way of being. And in Irish tradition, the waters of this world come from a single well in the Otherworld below.

John Moriarty said, "For us to learn to speak is to learn to say: 'our river has its source in an Otherworld well,' and anything we say about the hills and anything we say about the stars is a way of saying 'A Hazel grows over the Otherworld well our river has its source in.'"[2]

Within this framework, there is no distinction between physical and metaphysical geography. The dark world beneath our feet from which the wild waters come, from which the elemental essence of our being is drawn and to which it returns when we die, is not another dimension or another reality but a place, just like a hollow hill or an ocean or the surface of the moon or the cold black space between stars. Traditionally, the well is associated with the headwaters of the Bóinne, the river on Earth that mirrors the river of stars we call the Milky Way (known in Irish as Bealach na Bó Finne—the Way of the White Cow), which some say is the path souls travel on their journey between lives and worlds.

Sorcerer and folklorist Robin Artisson, whose work translates elements of the traditional Irish, Scottish, Cornish, Breton, and Welsh Fayerie or Faerie Faith into the context of the spiritual ecology of contemporary North America, writes that the unseen world "is not separate from or 'beyond' this world. It is deeply resident inside the world that we sense. It is an interior dimension to sensual things, a dimension that it just as natural as anything else we encounter with our senses."[3]

The unseen world is the darkness of the womb and of the grave and of the oceans from which life emerged and the emptiness from which the first matter and energy emerged. In the Irish mythos, it is the place to which the Tuath Dé, the Tribe of the Gods, the people who had brought magic and knowledge from the north and learned to work with and change the flows of wind and water, returned when they left this world, departing from a burial mound at the mouth of the Bóinne. It is that dimension of being where the infinite flows into the particular. Holy places and wild places, within ourselves and in the world, are where we can most easily meet that boundary. And sometimes we can cross it—but not without great risk.

In that Otherworld, the oldest creature in the world—the ancestor of all Salmon—swims in the well, eating the nuts that fall from the Hazel trees whose branches spread over the well from which the rivers flow, taking in all the wisdom the Hazel drew from the soil of that Otherworld and carrying it into our own. The Salmon of life within us is a descendant of that Salmon that knew the waters of that Otherworld. Wild water welling up from the ground brings a reminder of that world and our relation to it, and it can bring a new infusion of life or carry someone more smoothly toward death. The Salmon has long been connected with the health of the body and the health of the land in Irish tradition.

Naturalist and folklorist Niall Mac Coitir writes:

The salmon was regarded in Irish folk belief as the epitome of good physical and mental health, and the phrase sláinte an bhradáin ("the salmon's health") was synonymous with robust good health. Indeed, every person was said to have an internal "salmon of life" in his or her body, which overexertion could cause to be expelled, resulting in death if it were not immediately restored.[4]

What does it mean to see the life force flowing through someone's body as a Salmon swimming through the rocks and waters and tree roots and rivers and vast seas of an internal landscape? To begin with, it conjures up a visceral sense of flowing motion. A human pulse is like a Salmon swimming with the rhythmic rippling movement of its silvery muscular body.

Salmon swim upstream from the ocean to their spawning places in forest streams to give life to another generation. Unlike Pacific Salmon, who die right after they spawn, some adult Atlantic Salmon make it back to the sea alive, but some die of exertion on one leg or the other of their journey. Overexertion would leave a Salmon stranded on the rocks of a stream. Spending the life force unwisely would leave a person exhausted, unable to continue to move with the once smooth flow of life and in danger of death—an ubiquitous condition in contemporary society, a rare and serious one in precolonial Ireland.

The life and death of the Salmon was also deeply connected with the life and death of the land. Until the sixteenth century, most of the west of Ireland was covered with forests of Oak, Birch, Hazel, and Yew. In 1585, British officials ordered the cutting of the forests of the province of Munster to deprive rebels of a place to hide, clear land for English plantations, and provide timber for the British navy and merchant marine, which would soon begin the colonization of North America in earnest. Much of Ireland's remaining forest was cleared in the early years of the Industrial Revolution to fuel the furnaces of British factories.

When Salmon died of exhaustion or fell prey to Otters or Ospreys or Eagles or Herons, their carcasses would wind up on the riverbanks and be dragged into the forest by scavengers, nourishing the soil. In turn, the trees growing in soil fed by the bodies of Salmon filtered water through their roots and staved off sedimentation, keeping the streams clean for the Salmon who survived the spawning run and the Salmon being born in their waters. When the forests were cleared, the Salmon suffered. When the Salmon suffered, the soil suffered. When the soil suffered, the people suffered.

So to understand someone's life force as a Salmon is also to understand the person's health as bound up with the health of the forest, the health of the waters, the health of the land. The only way to experience the "health of the Salmon" is to live in a world where Hazelnuts fall into streams fed by underground springs and rainwater, where life can be led fluidly, and when at last life is done and you are floundering on the rocks, your body goes to feed the land that fed you.

When the streams filled with Salmon are lost, we need to go to the wells fed by ancient springs to recover the memory of the ways of being the Salmon and the forests taught to the people. The wild waters that rise from these wells have spent hundreds of years underground, and as they make their way back to the surface, they filter through soils infused with the chemical traces of roots and leaves and flowers and fruit that dissolved back into the earth when they died. In places where the water filters through peat, they carry the aromatic molecules of forests and fields that existed thousands of years ago. These wild waters are medicine from the time of our ancestors, carrying the memory of a different world.

We are watery creatures, our awareness fed by the streams of our senses. The waters of this world and of the Otherworld are also mirrored by our own inner waters—our blood and our interstitial fluids that carry chemical, kinetic, electrical, and photic signals through our bodies. In many cultures, water has long been associated with our emotions, our dreams, and our unconscious knowings. The late neuroscientist Candace Pert famously asserted that the body is the unconscious mind and that our hormones—the water-soluble molecules of our chemical signaling systems—are molecules of emotion. (Their fat-soluble chemical cousins, the neurotransmitters, travel across neural synapses, regulating electrical flows.) It is at this level of being that we viscerally understand and directly experience our relationship with all life.

Water, by its very nature, is fluid, malleable, and receptive. As a universal solvent, it tends to dissolve the boundaries between things. When it is still, it becomes a mirror. Moriarty writes that it was at the Otherworld Well that he "learned that being human was a habit. It could be broken."[5] By going to the wellspring of all life, it becomes possible to remember our connection with all things. The waters of our bodies are reminded of all the channels they have flowed through, all the forms they have known. Turning within, we see that the waters are portioned out through three cauldrons within us. Let us look now to those cauldrons.

There were forests here once
where now there is only limestone
and brush and thin soil;
the waters of the well
remember flowing
through roots of Oak and Fern
and earth that knew
the footsteps
of Deer and Fox and Hare
before the time
of the long gun
and the axe.
Macha told me
to bring my people home.
But I do not know
who my people are
and the distant forests
of home
are aflame.
So, I hang the tine
of the antler
of a Stag
from the Hawthorn
by the well
and Brighid leads me
up the hill
to the grave of
an gaiscíoch
na Poblacht
inscribed in Gaeilge
in 1922.

Beneath him
lie the bones
of chieftains
and kings
buried beneath
the mound
that the waters
might carry them
back to the arms
of their wild lover,
this land.
I hear her voice
and I am undone:
priest of a burning forest
bard of a language I've lost
King of dry bones
who will embrace
this body
when I am gone?
What river
will carry
me home?

3

The Three Cauldrons

Earth, water, and fire come together in the cauldron where life begins, and as we emerge from that cauldron, our choices determine the way we mediate their interactions, shaping our lives. My Irish ancestors understood the waters of our being to be held by three cauldrons warmed by three fires within the body. Understanding the nature of those three cauldrons can guide us in cultivating health.

What we know about the three cauldrons we have gleaned from a seventh-century poem, written in Old Irish, preserved in a sixteenth-century manuscript and attributed to the Bronze Age poet Amergin. Amergin was the bard of the tribe of Celts who first sailed to Ireland from Galatia, taking the land from the Tuath Dé, the Tribe of the Gods, who would become the Faerie people, the Daoine Sidhe, when they retreated into the dark, watery Underworld. Amergin gained sovereignty by courting the spirit of the land with poetry that spoke of his unity with all things—proclaiming that he had been a Hawk flying over cliffs, a Salmon swimming swiftly, a Stag with antlers of seven tines, a drop of dew gleaming in the sun.

"The Cauldron of Poesy" speaks of the nature and origin of poetry, which was connected with creation, destruction, and transformation in ancient Irish culture, and which he spoke of as arising from what is cooked in three cauldrons within the body: the Cauldron of Incubation, which is upright within us when we are born, the Cauldron of Motion, which starts off turned on its side but can become upright if we move in good ways in response to the joys and sorrows of life, and the Cauldron of Wisdom, which is inverted when we are born, pouring down blessings on us, but becomes upright when we attain an ecstatic state, from which we pour blessing out into the world. The Cauldron of Incubation is the birthplace of the Animal Self and one place where that self flows together with the God Self; the Cauldron of Motion can be seen as the meeting place of the Animal Self and the Human Self; and the Cauldron of Wisdom is the seat of the God Self that gives inspired expression through the ways in which the Animal Self experiences infinity and union giving rise to the emotion and rhythm of poetry. My favorite modern translation of the poem was done by Erynn Rowan Laurie, a poet and scholar who has played an important role in the Celtic Reconstructionist movement—where I quote from the text here, I quote from her translation.[1]

The Cauldron of Incubation holds the primal essence of who we are and who we will become. Amergin describes it as having "been taken by the Gods from the mysteries of the elemental abyss." It is the place where life begins, where watery potential is distilled into solid form. It is also the place where poetry's power to create and destroy is born—from it there "pours forth a terrifying stream of speech from the mouth."[2] I think here of the potent energy at the root in tantric traditions that rises along the spine, becoming the kundalini.

Most modern commentators and practitioners locate the Cauldron of Incubation in the belly, but for me, its name, its role as the place where the waters of life first enter into and become our being, and its place as the root of our primal poetic impulse all suggest the pelvis, which, in its form, is also more similar to a cauldron. I associate it with the root chakra and the sacral plexus in Westernized understandings of Vedic models of the body and with the function of the kidneys in Chinese medicine. I experience it as white, the color of starlight and bones and a color Celtic cultures have long associated with the Otherworld. Robin Artisson explores this connection at length in his book *An Carow Gwyn*. He connects whiteness with the pallor of death and hence with the realm of the ancestors.

In the pulse, I feel what is happening within the Cauldron of Incubation in the quality of the flow of blood across the third position on the wrist, the one associated with the kidneys in Chinese pulse diagnosis. And I feel the influence of events there on other organs and on the body as a whole at the third depth, the bone depth, which in Chinese pulse diagnosis tells us the material condition of the organ in question.

It is the place where formlessness moves into form, where we strike the balance between structure and flow. Herbalist Subhuti Dharmananda writes:

> First, there is essence, the intertwining of yin and yang that makes up all things. It has—this time—manifested as a human, the ultimate meeting of heaven (yang) and earth (yin). The essence, as a manifestation from earlier existence through the continuing cycle of death and rebirth, gains its new chamber, the kidney, which retains it and allows it to slowly emerge in form. From this precious chamber sprouts the skeleton, and within the spine, the spinal cord and brain, and from the brain the retina and hearing mechanism. Within the bones is the marrow which generates blood. Also from the kidney emerges the reproductive organs, so as to help assure another part of the linkage between earlier existence and later existence.[3]

The yang is that which seeks expression, and the yin is the living substance through which it manifests. The kidney yang is the fire that heats the Cauldron of Incubation; the kidney yin is the water within the cauldron.

We do need structure as well as flow. We are rivers held in by strands of protein and just enough minerals that we can stand upright and dance. To understand the nature of that structure, we turn to Brighid's dark twin, who presides over the dark months to come and is known by several names across Ireland and Scotland and the islands off their coasts: Bone Mother. Cailleach Béara. Nicnevin.

In Gaeilge traditions, she is the dark bride the land becomes at Samhain. Here, the north wind is her breath. The mountain range that shelters the lake where my house is mirrored is her spine, running south to Georgia and north and east to Ireland and Scotland.

If Brighid is the flowing water and the bright dancing flame, Cailleach Béara is the cold solidity of the earth that holds our ancestors' bones, the darkness of the womb and the grave. In Wales, she is Cerridwen, whose cauldron of death and rebirth is also associated with the power to shape-shift—a power that arises from our understanding that the water and proteins and minerals and fats that become our bodies had life as other bodies as well.

In the Irish tradition, that power of understanding comes from eating the body of the Salmon of Wisdom or eating the Hazelnuts that fall into the well where the Salmon dwells and the river has its source. Erynn Rowan Laurie has uncovered interesting evidence that these may be oblique references to the sacramental use of the *Amanita muscaria*, the iconic red and white mushroom of Northern European folklore. I have wondered myself, drawing more from inspiration and vision than from scholarship, if the *Psilocybe semilanceata* mushroom, the Liberty Cap mushroom, which grows in Cattle and Sheep pastures across Ireland and Britain, may have filled a similar role.

On both sides of the North Atlantic, Samhain, the time of Cailleach Béara's coronation, is the season of the Deer hunt and the culling of the Cattle herd. Throughout the winter my ancestors nourished themselves with the meat harvested at Samhain, and they broke open the bones and cooked them in great cauldrons over fires of driftwood and peat, often with seaweed gathered from the rocky shores.

In the season when the Cailleach Béara rules, we spend long nights in the shadow, confronting what we did not face in the bright light of day. Sometimes, in the darkness, we are stripped as bare as the Oak and the Birch in the winter. In such times, I remember the wise words shared by the doorkeeper in a North American ceremony, not unlike those of my ancestors, where we prayed all night for the rising of the sun: If you use your muscles to hold yourself up through the night, you will grow tired and sore. Instead, rest into your bones and let them support you.

In Chinese medicine, the kidney is the reservoir of our ancestral inheritance and the mother of the bone. That ancestral essence, the *jing,* is a watery thing that calcifies into solid form as we come together in the womb and as we grow in the world. It is also the source of the sexual fluids that carry and transmit our genetic inheritance.

We are learning that bone is a complex endocrine organ that evolved to help us escape from danger. When we sense danger, our bones release osteocalcin, a protein that acts as a hormone and initiates our stress response. It is worth noting that it does this not by directly signaling the adrenals to release cortisol and adrenaline, but by shutting down the parasympathetic function of the autonomic nervous system, letting our bodies know that it is time to stop rebuilding and repairing themselves and switch into survival mode. We come back to ourselves and each other by settling into our bones.

Recent archaeological discoveries suggest that storing Deer bones to sustain the tribe through lean times is one of the oldest human practices. A practice as old as simmering those bones and gathering to tell the stories and sing the songs that remind us who we are. Songs and stories are prayers chanted over the soup that will tell the molecules of the dissolving bones what form to take as they transmute from animal bone to human flesh.

Chinese medicine teaches that stress, worry, and struggle deplete the kidney yin, the primal material source of bone. Broths made from roots and animal bones are one of the oldest medicines for replenishing that essence—foods harvested in autumn that sustain us through winter. There is profound medicine in these bones themselves: their collagen and their minerals help us restore our own skeleton and the collagen of our own fascia, which gives us structure as well. Sweet-tasting roots hold the energy the plant sent down into the earth, storing that energy for the months when it would be harder to gather energy from the sun—roots that reach down to subterranean water. These roots, many of them the same polysaccharide-rich mucilaginous roots that I spoke of above, help us rebuild ourselves. Solomon's Seal and Shatavari roots are associated with replenishing the sexual fluids as well, though I personally speculate that their role as aphrodisiacs may have at least as much to do with their moistening the fascia, making us more receptive to touch and presence.

Chinese medicine traditionally uses the velvet Deer scrape from their antlers and the spring pollen of the Pine to nourish the fire at the root that moves the waters we replenish with the sweet, moistening herbs— hence their modern popularity among weight lifters, who are trying to build new tissue from the elements of life, and their reputation for increasing libido, which ultimately is just the life force itself. Scots Pine was a popular herb in springtime beers in Scotland before seventeenth-century cultural shifts turned beer from a brew frequently made with aphrodisiac, stimulant, and mildly mind-altering ingredients to a sedative and libido-reducing drink made with Hops. (Stephen Buhner goes into this at length in his book *Sacred and Herbal Healing Beers*.) Pungent, aromatic roots like those of Osha, Angelica, and even Ginger can also stimulate the fire that warms the Cauldron of Incubation. When the fire has all but died out, the intense heat of Wormwood can rekindle its spark. Gently warming Damiana, which brings blood flowing to the pelvis, helps to connect the Cauldron of Incubation with the Cauldron of Motion.

If the Cauldron of Incubation cannot hold on to energy, especially if there is too much urination or too much discharge of sexual fluids, then astringent herbs—the herbs that make your mouth pucker when you taste them—will be indicated. If you ask most people what quality they associate with the astringent taste, they will tell you that astringent herbs and foods are drying.

The first sensation we usually experience when we taste something astringent is a puckering of the tissues of the mouth, followed by a decrease in salivation. The puckering, not the dry sensation itself, is the keynote here. The puckering is the result of the fibers of the skin and muscle tissues binding together more tightly, which, in turn, locks in moisture, preventing it from being lost through secretion. Astringents separate things and give them structure by reinforcing boundaries. This is true of thoughts and emotions as well as of physical fluids—though we'll explore the former more when we discuss the Cauldron of Motion.

Astringents are often called tonics in old literature because they restore tone to tissues. This way of viewing tonification is reflected in our modern concept of muscle tone and muscle definition. When muscles grow weak, their fibers grow farther apart, and they begin to sag. They become less visible and less palpable beneath the skin, and they become less able to do their work. If you want your muscles to grow stronger, you carefully injure them by overloading them, causing small tears, which, when repaired, become areas where the muscle fibers are denser and more closely bound together. As muscle tone increases, muscle definition increases—the muscle becomes more recognizable by sight and touch and more clearly differentiated from the tissues around them.

Unfortunately, you cannot use astringent herbs as a substitute for exercise to increase muscle tone. The one thing that we do know increases resting muscle tone is strengthening the connection between each muscle and the brain through conscious focus on contracting and relaxing each muscle. However, some astringent herbs will help you keep from leaking life force, giving you more energy and stamina when you do exercise, especially when combined with herbs that light the fire at the root. Schisandra (*Schisandra chinensis*), the Ginseng cousin called Eleuthero, and Damiana are a favorite combination of mine here.

Misunderstandings of what the old texts mean when they speak of tonification have led to misunderstandings of herbs. When people read in old texts that Goldenseal is a "mucus membrane tonic," they tend to assume that means it is something you should take every day to improve general mucus membrane health. What the old texts actually mean is that Goldenseal is a mucus membrane astringent. When the mucus becomes thin and runny, Goldenseal helps check its flow.

So we can best understand astringent herbs as herbs that create boundaries against the secretion, flow, and infiltration of fluids by binding tissue fibers more closely together. Chinese medicine traditionally uses Schisandra, the five-flavor berry, to prevent the leakage of jing. Sumac in North America and the Middle East and Rowan in Ireland and Britain have an astringency and a tartness similar to those of Schisandra (though they lack its sweetness, bitterness, and hint of peppery heat) and can be used in similar ways to strengthen the container of the Cauldron of Incubation. All three have associations with the Stag and the hunt, suggesting stamina and focused awareness. All of the plants of the Rose family are astringent, with the plants of the *Rubus* genus—Raspberry, Blackberry, Salmonberry, Thimbleberry, and so on—with their three-leafed structures that suggest the form of the pelvic musculature, having a special affinity for this lower cauldron. Blackberry root is the most astringent of the *Rubus* medicines and is my go-to medicine whenever someone is losing fluids quickly.

Oak bark is profoundly astringent and was traditionally used to tan leather. The solidity of the Oak and its ability to draw down lightning and survive the lightning strike are deeply connected with its traditional associations with kingship in Celtic cultures—pointing to the role of king as protector but also to the role of the king as the one who draws down light and fire from the heavens to give new life to the land. Mushrooms proliferate around the Oak in the wake of a lightning strike.

Taoist medicine, which had its origins in the same time as the Vedic medicine and tantric science that the people who would become known as Indo-Europeans carried across a continent and an ocean to Ireland in the Neolithic, speaks of our lives being a river of destiny—what we inherit from the ancestors is the water, and the pull of the planets on those waters creates motion and flow—as does the way we move in the world. It is Earth that gives us structure. It is the fires of the sun melting the snow that gives movement and force.

The Cauldron of Motion is the place where the body distills its experience of the world, of the joys and sorrows of life. It is the seat of sensation, which Wilhelm Reich described as the bridge between the ego and the outer world, that gives rise to emotion, which Reich described as the movement of the organism in response to sensation, and thus the place from which we move, speak, and act in the world.[4]

All activity, physical and mental, requires the flow of oxygenated blood to our tissues. The Cauldron of Motion is the seat of that innate intelligence that guides this flow in response to inner and outer events. When we are in a state of health, this flow is free and rhythmic, like good poetry. It is reflected in health in a free and easy flow at the middle depth of the pulse, referred to in Chinese pulse diagnosis as the blood level, which reflects what is happening with our organs at a functional level. I experience it as red.

This corresponds in contemporary biomedicine with the concept of heart rate variability. The heart is not a mechanical pump with a single, regular, repeating, staccato rhythm, but a drum whose rhythm shifts and changes in response to our experience of the world. The best predictor of cardiac health and overall health is heart rate variability, the ability of the heart to shift fluidly from one rhythm to another, which tracks closely with the strength and clarity of the signals flowing across the vagus nerve that facilitates communication between the brain and every internal organ except the adrenal glands. The best way to restore or maintain heart rate variability is to walk mindfully in a forest, inhaling the exhalations of its plants, and with them the subtle signals contained in their release of aromatic compounds that the body recognizes as an invitation to connection.

Our perception of the world plays a role in guiding the rhythm and flow of our blood. When we feel safe, embodied, and connected, we are responsive to the world around us. The "Cauldron of Poesy" tells us that state is a result of a healthy turning of the Cauldron of Motion, inspired by the true joy that comes from intimate connection with the human, the wild, or the divine, or with great art, and by distilling the truths revealed by sorrow. In such a state, we are physically open, and we allow what stirs within us to be expressed freely in our movement and our communication. Fear closes us, creating constriction that can either cut off the flow altogether or lead to a building of pressure as intense forces press against strong barriers, which we will explore thoroughly in the next chapter.

Physical motion gets our blood and lymph flowing, which allows us to move through our experiences. Blood carries oxygen and hormones to our tissues. Lymph carries metabolic waste out of the tissues and is moved by the pressure created on lymphatic vessels by compression through exercise that contracts the muscles—or through massage or immersion in water.

When the circulation is deficient, we become cut off from awareness of some parts of our bodies (something exacerbated by constriction) and eventually begin to lose adequate blood flow to the brain. Hot herbs like Cayenne and Rosemary and herbs like Prickly Ash and Devil's Club, which create sharp sensations on the tongue (their spines are an interesting signature here), can bring us into sudden, sharp awareness, quicken the heartbeat, and send blood flowing more forcefully and swiftly through the body, especially when combined with an herb that removes the tension constricting the flow, like Lobelia. Warming herbs like Ginger, Cinnamon, Cardamom, Basil, and Sage provide gentler support for keeping blood and awareness flowing. Yarrow has the unique and mysterious ability to, as Matthew Wood says, guide the proper flow of the blood, preventing both clotting and hemorrhaging.

Fear can cause a sudden increase in the heart rate. Often this is associated with the release of histamine—a compound people best know through its association with allergies. Histamine serves multiple functions. As an immune factor, it signals the body to increase its local inflammatory response in the tissues where it is released to fight off infection and repair damage; and as a neurotransmitter, it serves to create and consolidate negative memories so that we will avoid being injured in the same way again and respond strongly if we feel something similar to that previous injury. It also stimulates an anxious response in the amygdala, which may partially explain the strong association that is being established between high histamine levels and addiction. Histamine will generate heat and redness. The leaves and flowers of many plants of the Rose family, especially Hawthorn, Rose, and Peach, are tremendously helpful in calming the physiological and emotional hyperreactivity that are associated with histamine releases.

Reishi mushrooms and their North American cousins of the *Ganoderma* genus have a long history of being used to calm the spirit, as well as a recent history of showing a remarkable capacity for modulating inflammatory immune responses. I have found that—over time for most people, and instantly for a few—Reishi can help bring a profound sense of stillness. Matthew Becker speaks of Reishi's capacity to "pull trauma from tissues." I experience this as a kind of metabolization of experiences and memories, analogous to the support Reishi provides for the liver's work of clearing physiological toxins and metabolic waste. There is an interesting signature present here. Reishi spreads its white mycelium through the wood of old trees, slowly breaking that wood down, bringing forth the red fruiting body of the mushroom, which releases golden spores into the wind. Wood holds the memory of the experience of the tree, as evidenced by the way we can read the history of a tree's life by looking at the rings within its trunk that mark each year of its growth, so Reishi is metabolizing the tree's experience—the same thing it does for us. The red of the fruiting body suggests the blossoming of life, and the golden spores dispersed on the wind suggest the luminous wisdom of a life well lived being passed on to others. The white of the mycelium, similar in form and function to our nerves, suggests consciousness reaching into the world of things past, those things to which blood no longer flows.

Schisandra, traditionally used as a meditation aid in China, combines beautifully with Reishi to calm an agitated heart. I think of Schisandra as an astringent of consciousness, gathering scattered and wandering flows of thought and emotion back inward to the heart. You could say that it helps plug leaks in all three cauldrons.

When agitation brings sudden, intense emotion to the surface, I rely on bitter Mint family plants to help draw the flow of blood and awareness down lower into the body. The bitter taste is profoundly grounding, and Mint family plants, like Rose family plants, tend to be good at calming excess heat without smothering the healthy heat of vitality. Lemon Balm is indicated when agitation brings sudden flashes of anger.

Motherwort is indicated when agitation brings sudden tears. If a person shows a tendency to weep himself into exhaustion, I will add to Motherwort's grounding bitterness the gentle cooling and subtle astringency of Rose—which will slow the tears without suppressing them.

Lack of motion—mental, physical, and emotional—can make the inner waters stagnant. We find ourselves stewing in the same neurotransmitters and hormones, ruminating on grievances and sorrows, reproducing the same emotions, which leads us to release more of the same hormones and neurotransmitters and to continue stewing in them. We also find ourselves more susceptible to outside influences, be they other people's thoughts and emotions that linger with us or actual chemical influences from an increasingly toxic world. Sometimes we need medicines and rituals of purification.

Large segments of our culture often conflate and confuse purification with purging and punishing the body—something not surprising when we consider that, whether we attend church or not, and whatever we ourselves believe, the culture of the United States and the culture of global capitalism it gives rise to are shaped by a version of Christianity that views the body and its earthly desires and pleasures as corrupt and sinful. These cultural forms are marked by the alternation of periods of gluttony with periods of severe deprivation, and periods of ignoring accumulating physical and emotional toxicity with harsh, cathartic cleanses for a body we either consciously or unconsciously view as dirty and sinful, especially in the United States, where a Puritan strain runs through the culture. New Age fixation on ascension and pure light, misunderstandings and misappropriations of Vedic and tantric concepts by North American yoga enthusiasts, colonics and extreme laxatives, all are rooted in a paradigm that seeks purification through discipline and punishment even though their language and their surface concepts are different from those of the fire-and-brimstone Puritanism of the seventeenth-century Massachusetts Bay Colony. This is not what I mean when I speak of purification.

Robin Artisson gives my favorite description of what purification means in the context of an animist worldview: "Purification is never about cleaning your 'gross human self' of some kind of moral stain, nor of separating yourself from any aspect of your humanity. It's simply about removing potential powers acting on you that hinder your work."[5]

Those influences acting on us can include the influence of neurotransmitters and hormones that were appropriate to another time and place but not to the one we are in here and now—both those that we discussed above that create heightened states of reactivity and those that move us in the opposite direction, toward grief and despair.

Orientation within time depends in part on connection with seasonal cycles. As my friend and teacher Cornelia Benavidez recently reminded me, people around the world have always come together to observe the seasonal changes in the sun, the moon, and the stars. Such times were marked by shared work of planting or harvesting or hunting, followed by feasting and celebration. They were also times of ritual and prayer, when people would tap into their own bodies' sense of the changes afoot in the world and use the momentum of the winds and the currents and the shifts in the lives of plants and animals and the land and water themselves to remember how to create the same kinds of change in their inner worlds. (In chapter 7, I will introduce you to my own seasonal ritual cycle, aligned with the four great fire festivals of my Irish ancestors: Samhain in late autumn, Imbolc in late winter, Bealtaine in late spring, and Lughnassadh in late summer.)

Ritual resets the rhythm of the heart and the blood, which is partly why drumming, singing, and dancing are some of the oldest ritual techniques in the world. In the earliest rituals we have evidence of, people donned animal skins and moved like the animals in the world around them, reminding the Animal Self how to be an animal in the season the world was entering. Most martial arts hold versions of this ancient knowledge of using movement in precise ways to change and focus consciousness and guide action in ways that are at once swift and fluid.

The rituals that connect us with the life cycles of the other-than-human beings around us also serve to orient us to cycles of birth and death in ways that allow us to face our own mortality and shift our identification from our individual bodies to the body of the world. It is worth noting that the three therapies that seem to be most effective for treating the anxiety and depression associated with the diagnosis of a terminal disease are gardening, spending time in the wilderness, and exploring the inner wilderness of the unconscious with psychedelics—all of which would have served a similar role for our ancestors going back at least to the origins of agriculture in the Neolithic and perhaps to the tending of populations of wild plants by humans and other hominins long before then. Our earliest evidence of the existence of death rituals comes from a bouquet of Yarrow flowers buried with the body of a Neanderthal child in what is now Iraq. I am moved and inspired by the thought of an ancient tradition of—honoring the dead with the offering of a plant that facilitates the healthy flow of blood in the body when it is alive.

In an era of electric lights and reliable indoor heat (for those who can afford them) and a global economic system that keeps the same foods reliably on the supermarket shelves of wealthy nations throughout the year, we are no longer immersed in those rhythms unless we make a conscious choice to be. Our disconnection with the sun in and of itself creates major disruptions in our internal rhythms. We are beings of light and darkness as much as we are beings of earth, air, fire, and water.

Gil Hedley points out that the cranium is translucent around the eyes, allowing light to reach the pineal gland, which plays a central role in regulating sleep and dreaming. Our skin is translucent, too, allowing light to penetrate into our fascia. He explained this to an interviewer:

When the Periodic Chart of the Elements was being developed, the discovery of the elements was a process involving light. The elements have characteristic absorption and emission spectra which can be discerned by interpretation with a spectroscope. Whether carbon, hydrogen, nitrogen, oxygen, or the rest, the elements alone and in combination emit light. The human body, comprised of these elements, is a light emitting, light absorbing phenomenon, and this is an aspect of our human anatomy that we might do well to consider in our quest for self understanding and health. I am fond of saying that "the human body" is not limited by the boundaries of our skin. We are all part of one human body, and the sun is a shared organ, our "master gland."[6]

Victor Anderson spoke of the sun as the god of our solar system because its light and heat and gravity and electromagnetic winds shape everything that happens here. The identification of seasonal affective disorder and the success of treatments for it—vitamin D-3, full spectrum light, and that most solar of plants, St. John's Wort, which blooms at Midsummer, when the sun is at its peak—have brought some awareness to the role of the sun in mental health. Just as important as sunlight, though, is darkness, and the dreaming we do within that darkness.

Traditionally, in many parts of the world, the dark months of the year were a time of telling certain stories around the fire that could only be told after the first frost or the first snow and the long nights of dreaming. Storytelling and dreaming are both ways that we metabolize experiences and emotions in ways that give us just enough removal from the original situation to be able to process them more fully: stories allow us to see someone else go through experiences we might have shared, letting us recontexualize those experiences without completely reliving them. Dreams allow us to repeat and complete sensations and emotions that remain unresolved from waking life. We are also more receptive to the whispers of the Otherworld when we are dreaming. The Irish year begins in darkness at Samhain, mirroring the way we emerge into the world only after gestating in the dark waters of the womb.

Sleep is also the time when our liver does most of its work of metabolizing the hormones that have circulated through our blood throughout the day, as well as anything the body doesn't want to assimilate or reassimilate. Chinese medicine likens the work of the liver to a cleansing wind. Subhuti Dharmananda writes:

The liver is the source of wind. The wind disperses the water vapors and clouds and lets spaces develop, through which the great yang, the sun, can shine and the wood can grow. The penetrating and reflecting light enters through the eyes and the images then restrain or agitate the wind.[7]

Wind is always in motion, and this clearing and cleansing of the liver is also a function of the Cauldron of Motion. The element of wood—the element of new growth in spring—is also housed in and associated with the liver in Taoist medicine. The wood yang is the ability to advance toward our goals; the wood yin is the ability to relax and withdraw. The quality of the liver's function is felt in the second position on the wrist (two fingers down from the scaphoid) in Chinese pulse diagnosis, and this is one of the ways I assess what is happening within the Cauldron of Motion. The deepest level of the pulse there tells me what impact processing past events has had on the liver, the middle depth tells me how the liver is processing the past right now, and the level closest to the surface tells me how the liver feels about what it is about to begin responding to.

Sleep and water are what the liver needs most—water to allow for flow, sleep to allow for time when the internal wind is not being influenced by new information pouring in through the eyes. The body perceives alcohol and most pharmaceuticals as toxins, which force the liver to work hard to process them; though sometimes purposeful poisoning is necessary to stop even more harmful processes, so pharmaceuticals are not universally unhealthy choices. But this additional work disrupts the liver's daily processing role, and since the liver's physical processing of hormones is integral to our emotional processing through dreaming, these toxins disrupt our emotional processing too.

Reishi is one of my favorite allies for helping people process things through dreaming. I learned about this years ago when someone came to me for panic attacks that had begun suddenly, in the wake of big life changes. I gave her a formula that included Reishi to settle the heart. She came back a few weeks later and said that the panic attacks were less frequent and that in her dreams she had been meeting with people she had unfinished business with and bringing old situations to resolution, so I continued her on that formula. A few weeks later she came back and said that everything was great, but that she was waking up feeling like she had done too much work in her dreams. So we took the Reishi out, and the dream meetings stopped. Later, she wanted to resume that dream work, so I added Reishi back in, and sure enough, the dreams returned.

For people who wake from dreams startled and agitated, I like to combine Reishi with Schisandra and Motherwort. When that waking is sudden and fearful, I give a single drop of Wormwood.

What we don't metabolize, we hold on to. Since communication within our bodies is facilitated by water and lipids conducting chemical and electrical signals, this tends to present in the form of stagnant, swampy conditions, with tissues bogged down with metabolic waste that blocks circulation.

Stifled emotions that are still fresh or are swiftly remobilized tend to present as anger, manic laughter, or the hot tears of sudden sorrow. Think of the heat you can feel beneath the surface of a compost pile, the heat of a continuous process that is blocked from finding its way out into the world. I treat these kind of resurfacing hot emotions the same way I treat hyperreactivity: with bitter, cooling Mints like Lemon Balm, Motherwort, and Skullcap; the cooling flowers of Rose and Hawthorn; and plants that release tension to allow the heat to flow through (something we will soon discuss at great length).

But some emotions, particularly grief, tend to settle into the watery places in the body, especially the lungs and the fascia. They bog us down and often have the dull, aching quality of rheumatic pains—your soul can feel the way an arthritic person's bones and joints feel just before a rainstorm. The body needs help clearing them. Bitter, warming, aromatic herbs can accomplish this well. Their bitterness stimulates the liver, the heat stimulates the circulation, and the aromatic quality opens and engages the mind and the senses.

In the early stages of such malaise, kitchen herbs like Basil, Rosemary, Onion, and Sage can be helpful, as can teas and steams of Evergreen needles. When I lived on the West Coast, I would always have fresh Red Cedar boughs present in the room when working with a grieving person and would encourage grieving people to burn dried Cedar leaves at home. Now that I am back in Maine, I use the needles, resin, and cones of White Pine for steams to open the lungs and move recent, fresh grief. Burning Frankincense can help raise the spirits in such times as well.

When grief has lingered longer, stronger medicines are needed. Most are roots that grow in damp places: Angelica, Elecampane, Eastern and Western Skunk Cabbage. They clear the grief held in the lungs and open the airways to allow the breath of life to enter again. Black Cohosh helps to ease this kind of stagnant depression by allowing the cerebrospinal fluid to detoxify the brain—when we stew in the same old neurotransmitters we stew in the same old emotions. Calamus relights the fire of expression, allowing us to burn through the fog and give voice to the deepest truths that rise up through us.

The folk medicine of disparate cultures throughout the world's northern latitudes long recognized the need to move the inner waters during the transitions between the dark and bright times of the year. The Birch sap that rises as spring approaches and spring greens like Dandelions, Cleavers, Violets, and Nettles were welcomed as foods that would "purify the blood" by helping the liver, the kidneys, and the lymph carry metabolic waste out of the body after long months of being confined indoors and eating heavy foods.

When autumn came, people would go through another round of purification so they would not be carrying so much heaviness that it would wear them down as they entered the dark of the year. From the Bronze Age into the late nineteenth century, people in Ireland, like their counterparts in North America, Scandinavia, and Siberia, would seek the aid of fire and darkness in preparing them for winter. In Ireland, people built peat fires in stone chambers and sealed up the entrance, staying inside for hours, coming out occasionally to plunge in water.

The name for this kind of chamber was *teach alais*—the sweathouse.

We have only nineteenth-century accounts to go on to understand the nature of this ritual. Those texts, written by English-speaking people describing what they heard and observed among people in the countryside, tell us that the sweathouses were mainly used to treat rheumatism and that women would occasionally put Kelp on the fire to aid their complexions.

Is it possible that the ritual had a deeper significance as well? I would say that it is almost certain that it did, though we will likely never know because people in an occupied country whose native language had been outlawed were unlikely to tell even sympathetic interviewers from the occupying culture about remnant ancestral spiritual practices. But everywhere else where such rituals are performed, they serve—or originally served—the purpose of spiritual purification. And where ritual forms are the same, ritual functions tend to be as well, at the very least, in the early forms of the ritual. Darkness has a way of turning the mind inward, and aromatic smoke like that of a peat fire puts people into a receptive state. Heat stirs the blood, and sweat helps release the memories the body holds. The Irish frame drum, the bodhrán, and the haunting sounds of *sean-nós* singing, the trance-based vocal style of Ireland's Gaeilge-speaking West, may have played a role in further facilitating shifts in consciousness that would allow access to the guidance of the Otherworld. It is also significant that this would have been a ritual of going naked into the darkness during the time of year when the ancestors and the Daoine Sidhe are said to walk most closely with us.

We know that the Irish had extensive contact with Scandinavian people, sometimes as adversaries and sometimes as trading partners, and they likely also had contact with the Indigenous peoples of the areas that are now New England and Canada's Maritime provinces. The Tuath Dé, the Tribe of the Gods, are said to have been people who left Ireland to go to the north and returned bearing magic and knowledge, which they took with them beneath the hollow hills, the ancient burial mounds, when they left this world. Later sages, poets, and saints were said to have sailed to lands far to the west and returned bearing the fruits of the visions they experienced there. Cross-pollination of ritual and medicinal techniques among all the people of northern latitudes seems more a certainty than a possibility.

All of this brings us to the nature of the third and final cauldron—the Cauldron of Wisdom. The Cauldron of Wisdom is inverted in us when we are born, and it remains inverted throughout most people's lives. Its waters are the waters of the infinite—just as in the Cauldron of Incubation, just as in the Otherworld Well. For most people, those waters flow down through the Cauldron of Motion, with more and more wisdom being retained as engaging joy and sorrow turns that middle cauldron more and more upright. Many people, however, never do the necessary work for the Cauldron of Motion to be turned from its initial position—tilted on its side—with the result that the water from the Cauldron of Wisdom spills out and is lost. I experience this cauldron as the electric blue of the sky just before dawn and as the center of the flame. It doesn't show up in the pulse directly, but I can often feel elements of its influence on the Cauldron of Motion in the layer of the pulse closest to the surface and in the first pulse position on the left wrist, the position just below the scaphoid, which is connected with the heart in Chinese pulse diagnosis.

Then there are the *filidh*, the poets (singular: *fili*) who turn the Cauldron of Wisdom upward and light a fire beneath it. Poetry was not just a form of personal expression in ancient Ireland, especially for the filidh. Erynn Rowan Laurie tells us:

> The word fili probably means "seer." The word derives from the Archaic Irish *weis* by way of the Insular Celtic word *wel*—which had the original imperative meaning "see!" or "look at!" and is related to the Irish verb *to be*. Their work included divination, blessing and blasting magic, creating praise poetry for their patrons, the preservation of lore and genealogies, and occasionally the rendering of judgments. *Cormac's Glossary* derives *fili* from "*fi*, 'poison' in satire, and li, 'splendor' in praise, and it is variously that the poet proclaims."[8]

Poetry is the language of the Human Self that comes closest to expressing the Animal Self's experience of its encounters with the living world, the Otherworld, and the divine. Its imagery invokes the presence of plants, animals, ancestors, and forces of nature. Its rhythm induces trance. Its sounds evoke emotion. A properly trained fili had the power to speak words that could heal or could harm and the power to write withering words that would take away the power of a corrupt or brutal chieftain or king. The greatest poetry speaks to all three selves and calls them into alignment. It comes from the root, out of the Cauldron of Incubation, moves upward through the Cauldron of Motion, and then, if the Cauldron of Motion is fully upright and all the conditions are right, it blazes up as a fire in the head that warms the Cauldron of Wisdom and pours forth as "a terrifying stream of speech from the mouth."

Such poetry emerges during a state of *imbas,* "poetic frenzy," cultivated through time in the wilderness, scrying (divinatory gazing) in lakes and wells, immersion in darkness, and other techniques of shifting consciousness. This may have included the ingestion of visionary medicines like the ones we will discuss in chapter 5. A fascinating, if highly speculative, book by Peter Lamborn Wilson called *Ploughing the Clouds* makes an intriguing case that the ancient Irish, like some other northern peoples, may have used the iconic red and white *Amanita muscaria* mushroom for ritual purposes. Erynn Rowan Laurie and Timothy White make a similar argument, more cautiously, in their essay "Speckled Snake, Brother of Birch." Among other things, they suggest that descriptions of filidh eating raw flesh from the mounds of the Daoine Sidhe may have been an oblique reference to harvesting and eating the mushroom—which, like Reishi, is the red, vital, fruiting body of a fungus that emerges from the white mycelium of an organism that feeds off dying roots and rotting leaves and other decaying matter. So to eat of the flesh of such a mushroom truly would be to partake of something of the Otherworld. (It also can be a good way to unintentionally become a permanent denizen of the Otherworld—*Amanita muscaria* is toxic at the wrong dosage or in the wrong preparation. Fledgling psychonauts would do well to stick with the gentler mushrooms of the *Psilocybe* genus that sprout up in pastures as Samhain approaches.)

Describing the state the filidh would enter, Laurie writes:

The translation of the word *imbas* as "poetic frenzy" is not an over-statement of the condition. This Celtic form of enlightenment is no gentle melding with the oneness of the universe. Instead, it is a passionate, sometimes uncontrollable engagement with the fabric of reality. The energies accessed when all the cauldrons are turned into their upright positions does indeed feel like fire flowing through the head, expanding, quickening, and burning, as when Amergin pro-claimed "I am a God who shapes fire for a head."[9]

This is the true definition of an ecstatic state. Though, as Amergin himself tells us, great and pure joy can lead to ecstasy; ecstasy is not joy, and while it has elements of bliss it also has elements of terror. The word *ecstasy* is derived from the Greek word *ekstasis,* which means "dis-placement, distraction, astonishment, entrancement." Navigating this state takes great skill and great focus.

Celtic traditions, both Gaelic traditions like those of Ireland and Scotland and Brythonic traditions like those of Cornwall, Wales, and Brittany, are full of warnings that encounters with the Otherworld, espe-cially encounters that occur at powerful places or powerful times of year, will render a person "mad, dead, or a poet." The training of the filidh prepared them to resolve madness into poetry before it could kill them. But to encounter the Otherworld was also to touch death and to be for-ever transformed in ways that may make you seem mad to the rest of the culture and will definitely make the rest of the culture seem mad to you.

The nature of such an encounter with the Otherworld is described by an Irish legend, the Vision of Óengus. Óengus Óg was the son of the Dagda, the "Good God," whose cauldron of plenty fed all of his people, and he was trained by Manannán Mac Lir, the powerful and mysterious god of wild waters who had already been in Ireland when the Tuath Dé arrived and who instructed them in magic, poetry, and music—which, from an ancient perspective, are really all one and the same. The Dagda made his home in an ancient burial mound at the mouth of the Bóinne. This mound would—through the clever wordplay Óengus learned from Manannán—become Óengus's home.

Later, this mound became the place where Manannán gathered the people when it was time for them to leave this world for the Otherworld. He divided the ancient burial mounds spread across Ireland, which are entrances to that realm, among the departing people as they became the Daoine Sidhe, the Faerie people, the People of the Mound. The Bóinne is the river that mirrors the Milky Way, and both have their source in the Otherworld Well.

It was in that mound, by that river—in the time when the Tuath Dé still lived and breathed as we do—that Óengus had a dream in which a woman of unearthly beauty appeared beside his bedside. When he went to reach for her hand, she vanished. When Óengus woke, an illness was upon him. He did not eat that day. That night he went to bed and dreamed the same dream. Nothing in his waking life could compare to the splendor of this vision. And so for two years, Óengus had this recurring dream. (It is also worth noting that all of these symptoms would be consistent with regular ingestion of *Amanita muscaria*, which might have been possible to do without getting even sicker in a time when people's livers were less challenged by environmental toxins, though it would never be wise from a mental health standpoint.)

Across cultures we see the same basic story repeated: A person's true vision awakens in dream. They cannot rest until they have understood how to integrate what they witnessed in that dream, and they become sick, often to the point of death. In the process, they wither away and die, go mad, or learn to view and experience the world in a new way, a way that perceives and weaves with the threads of time and space themselves. Mad, dead, or a poet, indeed.

Desperate to heal his son's illness, the Dagda sent people to search the land for the woman from his son's dream. He learned that her name was Caer Ibormeith and she lived in Connacht, a rocky province ruled by Queen Meadbh, who, like Manannán, had been in Ireland before the coming of the Tuath Dé and who often returned after their departure. Queen Meadbh was known for coming to test the worthiness of those who would be chieftains and kings by appearing to them as an old hag and asking them to make love to her. If they assented, she transformed into a young woman, and in the union with her, the man who would be king was wedded to the land. As we shall see shortly, like her queen, Caer treasured her sovereignty and tested her suitor's willingness to honor it.

Caer Ibormeith's name has great significance. *Caer* means "berry" in Irish Gaeilge (oddly, the same word means "fortress" in Welsh), and *ibormeith* refers to the Yew tree. The berries and leaves of the Yew are highly toxic, causing cardiac and respiratory failure—stilling the Cauldron of Motion. (Yes, as some of you may be aware, a substance from the Pacific Yew is used in treating some forms of breast cancer—but, remember, chemotherapy is an art of administering poison in precisely the right manner and dosage to kill cancer cells without killing the entire organism.) The tree itself is so ancient as to seem immortal. When it grows old, its branches become hollow, suggesting a passage to the Otherworld. When the tree becomes too heavy with age, it can split its trunk without risking disease or facture. It also has an interesting reproductive strategy: it chooses from year to year whether to grow reproductive structures we humans designate as masculine or feminine according to what its community needs, hence it is a shape-shifter. Because of these qualities, Yew is associated with ancestral magic and the magic of the dead—in other words, the powers of the Otherworld. It is for this reason that Yew trees are found in many church cemeteries across areas of Europe where Celtic tribes once lived. Those cemeteries were dug on ground already consecrated as burial grounds by the Indigenous cultures that lived there and blessed with the presence of the Yew.

Caer had strong magic of her own. When the Dagda tried to force her father to give her hand in marriage to Óengus, her father replied that he could not compel her to marry anyone, for her power was greater than his own. She had the power to transform from the form of a woman to that of a Swan or from the form of a Swan into that of a woman at Samhain. To court her, Óengus would have to meet her at the water's edge when Samhain came around again.

The Old Irish text, as translated by Jeffrey Gantz in his book *Early Irish Myths and Sagas*, tells us what happened the following Samhain.

> [Óengus] went to Loch Bél Dracon, and there he saw the three fifties of white birds, with silver chains, and golden hair about their heads. Oengus was in human form at the edge of the lake, and he called to the girl, saying "Come and speak with me, Cáer!" "Who is calling to me?" asked Cáer. "Oengus is calling," he replied. "I will come," she said, "if you promise me that I may return to the water." "I promise that," he said. She went to him, then: he put his arms round her, and they slept in the form of swans until they had circled the lake three times. Thus, he kept his promise. They left in the form of two white birds and flew to Bruig ind Maicc Oic [Óengus's habitation at the mouth of the Bóinne], and there they sang until the people inside fell asleep for three days and three nights.[10]

This part of the story is remarkable on several levels: in order to meet Caer in the fullness of her power, Óengus had to himself become a Swan. When they first made love, and when they traveled home, they did so in bird form. When they arrived, together they sang the incantations that put all present into the kind of deep sleep that was ritually used for the incubation of visions.

One thing that connects the filidh with the shamans of other cultures is that they wore cloaks made of feathers—and in the case of the filidh, those were cloaks of Swan feathers. A Swan travels three realms—the earth, the heavens, and the waters. Óengus's wedding was also an initiation.

I have been beautifully haunted by this story since childhood, when, as a precocious eight-year-old, I first read William Butler Yeats's liberally interpreted poetic retelling of the beginning of the story—"The Song of Wandering Aengus."[11] Yeats's original working title for his poem was "A Mad Song," which points to the thin, thin line between the visionary fervor of ecstatic frenzy and true psychosis. The poem begins with the words:

> *I went out to a hazel wood*
> *Because a fire was in my head.*

Every time I read those lines, I feel a spark of that fire leap into me. The fire in the head compels us to go into the forest to reconnect with the wholeness of who we are. To do that, we must first slip the constraints of this culture, and the madness those constraints can bring once the fire has begun to burn.

> *What wild spring rises through me?*
> *What strange fire burns in my heart?*
> *Though snow flutters like white moths on the wing*
> *and the rolling hills are sleeping Swans beneath a*
> *   starry sky*
> *the buds of the Cottonwood swell,*
> *the sap rises in the Maple and the Birch,*
> *and deep within a tight, tight bud*
> *the Apple blossom waits*
> *to send its scent*
> *to guide me home in springtime*
> *before the mountainside blooms.*

4

Mad, Dead, or a Poet

The ancient Greeks spoke of a wild man with the legs and horns of a goat who dwelt in the forests and hills beyond the city walls and the village edge. Sometimes when the wind was right, you could catch his strange music and his musky scent drifting through the air, calling you to a wild dance. They said that to encounter Pan was to risk madness, that his music induced *panikon,* which simply means "panic," in the hearts of villagers and the city folk.

Hidden beneath that warning is a deeper truth: you only experience panic if you resist the wild dance. You force your muscles to tense— but your Animal Self wants to move with the music. Your thwarted desire does not die down; it pushes against the tension, forcing the movement—and the amplification—of the fear you locked into your muscles when you decided to resist the call to dance.

In the Irish tradition we see those experiencing great violence and trauma fleeing to the wilderness for refuge. Most striking perhaps is the story of one of the last Pagan kings in Ireland, Suibhne Geilt, known in English as Mad Sweeney. (*Geilt,* Irish Gaeilge for "madness," is derived from the Proto-Celtic word *gʷeltis,* which means "wild." It is also the term for a class of ecstatic poets who spent time alone in the wilderness in order to be able to allow the fire in their heads to blaze freely.) To put the story in its simplest terms, Suibhne was cursed by a saint for fighting back against the construction of a Christian church on his family's sacred land. When next he went into battle, he was driven mad by the sounds of war and fled into the wilderness. In that time, Ireland was covered with great forests of Oak and Hazel, and Suibhne grew feathers and leapt from tree to tree.

When the madness passed through him, he came back from the forest and became a monk. Some of the greatest lyric poetry in the Irish language is written from the point of view of the elderly Brother Suibhne remembering his time in the forest. The late Irish poet and Nobel laureate Seamus Heaney captures better than anyone else writing in English the spirit of the original Gaeilge text. In one particularly striking passage, Sweeney, as Heaney calls him, describes how he forsook the call of the trumpet, sound of the hunt and of battle, for the trumpeting of the Stag, the great Red Deer, symbol of sovereignty and kingship in Pagan Ireland.[1]

> *I prefer the re-*
> *echoing of the belling of a Stag*
> *among the peaks*
> *to that arrogant horn.*
>
> *Those unharnessed runners*
> *from glen to glen!*
> *Nobody tames*
> *that royal blood,*
>
> *each one aloof*
> *on its rightful summit,*
> *antlered, watchful.*

The Irish word for Stag is *fia fierann,* which is related to the words *fiáin,* which means "wild," and *fear,* which means "man." The Red Deer is actually an Elk and the Red Deer Stag has the same bugling voice as the male North American Elk. The English call the Red Deer Stag the Roebuck. Pagan kingship in Ireland was rooted in being wedded to the land and carried the obligation to defend the vulnerable in the same way that the Stag protects the herd. I gained a visceral understanding of this when first I met the Red Deer.

In the forests and fields above Loch Léin in Killarney (Cuille Airne, "Church of the Blackthorn Berry"), in the shadow of the castle where the *taoisigh* (chieftains) of my clan lived, some of the last descendants of the original native herds of Red Deer live.

In autumn, the Red Deer Stags gather branches, Ferns, and moss to crown their antlers. In the time of rutting, and in the time of the Deer hunt, they engage in ritual combat. The Stag who emerges victorious becomes the locus of power within the herd, its protector.

In the weeks before the rutting season began, I traveled to the remnant forest those herds call home, seeking to understand the ways of my ancestors. I prayed beneath an Oak at the edge of a field, and then rounded the bend to a thicket, where a Stag came out to meet me— barrel-chested and with antlers as wide as my arm span. He raised his head high and cantered across the field—first showing his power, then trying to lead me away from the herd, and then circling it to mark a protective boundary.

I sat still, and soon he did too, resting beneath a tree while the does and the younger bucks grazed. In the way of the wild, when he knew his kin were safe, he relaxed into calm presence.

I understood then that it was the Stag who taught us what a chieftain was—not the other way around. This was the authentic expression of sovereignty that Suibhne tried to hold on to in the face of the model of leadership that came in with Christianity—a model that sought to make the king and the chieftain enforcers of the rigid laws in a book written in a distant desert, as interpreted by Latin-speaking theologians. The restriction imposed by those laws was an insult to Suibhne's soul, and his soul rebelled against that restriction, driving him into the wilderness.

There is an interesting parallel in the story of Mis, daughter of a king named Dair (*dair* is an Irish word for "Oak"), who was driven mad with grief when she found her father's severed head on the battlefield. She fled into the mountains that now bear her name and grew claws and long hair and defended her freedom ferociously. She was brought back to the world of humans by the patience, tenderness, and music of a harpist who went into the mountains to court her. Sharon Blackie retells the story beautifully in *If Women Rose Rooted*.

I have always found that when the life of this culture becomes too brutal and restricting for me, time in the forest allows my terror or rage or grief to have room to flow freely until, emptied of my pain, I can allow the scent of Spruce and Pine, the drumming of the Pileated Woodpecker, and the call of the Loons from the lake below to call me back to myself. I have known many veterans who have found healing from the ravages of war by spending time in the wilderness, outside the restrictions and expectations of the society that sent them to see and do and experience things that those at home do not want to know about.

In a lecture, John Moriarty said that a psychosis is bigger than the universe that contains it.[2] One way of dealing with that reality is to carefully and deliberately loosen the boundaries that the Human Self's beliefs place on the Animal Self's experiences, and then let the Animal Self have the space to run free. From Suibhne Geilt to John the Baptist, the wilderness has long been the refuge of those whose vision and passion could not be contained by the structures and strictures of society. Attempting to resist the call of such visions and stirrings courts even greater madness than following them.

Wilhelm Reich understood anxiety and trauma in similar terms— and saw them as endemic to modern life. Reich's teacher and mentor Sigmund Freud saw the human body as animated by the libido, the personal erotic drive. Eros in the original Greek sense referred to the drive to live. Freud saw the libido primarily in sexual terms, narrowly and literally defined. He believed that civilization depended on the taming and subjugation of this force and that a healthy culture was the result of the redirection of the libido.

Reich saw the libido manifested in a physical force, which he called orgone, which flowed through the body from the core to the periphery. He believed this energy was one and the same as sexual energy, but that its function was not limited to the realms we would define as "sexual." He saw this force, in fact, as the driving force of life itself, the "vegetative energy" that was expressed not only in the full and free expression of a liberated human being but also in the sprouting of a seed, the Dolphin's joyous leaping from the sea, the electricity of a lightning storm, the dance of the aurora borealis, the blazing of the sun, and the swirling life of the galaxy. He writes: "Since the life process and the sexual process are one and the same, it goes without saying that the sexual, vegetative energy is active in everything that lives."[3]

Reich shared his teacher's belief that this civilization as we know it depends on the subjugation of that erotic force, but he believed that repression was harmful. He saw that repression as something that created physiological tension that blocked the flow of orgone through the body and saw that obstruction as the root of most modern mental and physical illnesses. He understood anxiety as the consequence of upwelling energy in the body being blocked by tension and reanimating the fear that had created the tension in the first place.[4]

From a biological standpoint, our muscles constrict when we receive a signal from our limbic system—that ancient part of the brain that warns us when we face an impending threat. Our muscles tense to prepare to deliver or receive a blow or to run away. When the threatening situations we experience remain unresolved, as most of the stressful situations in contemporary life do, we remain constricted.

Tension serves not only to help us brace against experiences but also to neutralize, numb, or sequester sensory and emotional memories. Herbalist jim mcdonald notes that "tension or spasm in tissues impedes the flow of the circulation and the body's vital force."[5] Where blood flows, awareness goes. Where the flow of blood is cut off, so is awareness. Cutting off awareness by restricting blood flow is one of the body's brilliant strategies for helping us continue to act when we are in seemingly impossible situations. It prevents us from being completely awash in unbearable sensations and memories.

Reich observed the effects of chronic tension, and its impediment to the flow of the vital force in his patients:

> If the layer of rigidified conflicts were especially numerous and functioned automatically, if they formed a compact, not easily penetrable unity, the patient felt them as an "armor" surrounding the living organism. The armor could lie on the "surface" or in the "depth," could be "as soft as a sponge" or "as hard as a rock." Its function in every case was to protect the person against unpleasurable experiences. However, it also entailed a reduction in the organism's capacity for pleasure.[6]

Reich, who watched and spoke out against the rise of fascism in Europe before fleeing to the United States, saw that this armoring both reinforced and was reinforced by cultures of cruelty, violence, and rigid control:

> The character structure of modern man, who reproduces a six-thousand-year-old patriarchal authoritarian culture is typified by characterological armoring against his inner nature and against the social misery which surrounds him. This characterological armoring of the character is the basis of isolation, indigence, craving for authority, fear of responsibility, mystic longing, sexual misery, and neurotically impotent rebelliousness.[7]

If you cannot feel the pulsing of life at your own core, how can you feel the flow of life in a forest stream and understand that it is related to the flow of life within you? If you cannot feel your own sorrow or pain, how can you feel another's? Cutting off sensation cuts off empathy. Early in the Cold War, Robert Jay Lifton, a psychiatrist who worked with soldiers who had committed atrocities, coined the phrase *psychic numbing* to refer to the way in which the psyche fragments in order to keep the core persona from experiencing the horrors it is participating in. He later documented the ways in which psychic numbing can take place across entire societies, describing the ways in which people in the United States continued life as usual in the face of the threat of nuclear annihilation.[8] Buddhist psychologist, activist, and writer Joanna Macy has developed a repertoire of practices called "The Work That Reconnects" that seeks to reawaken and reintegrate the numbed parts of our psyches through meditation and rituals that reconnect us with the beauty and fragility of human and other-than-human life.[9]

No amount of psychic numbing can shut us down permanently and completely. When life, as it will, stirs within that armor and pushes against it, the armored person, who viscerally believes that his armor is the one thing protecting him from the world (and the world from his own instincts and desires), experiences profound anxiety. Reich saw that the solution to this was releasing that armoring, which would restore healthy flow to the system.

In many ways, Reich's approach aligns with ideas of traditional Western herbalism. Going back to the time of the ancient Greeks, Western herbal traditions have spoken of a vital force that animates the body and moves from the core to the periphery. These traditions have seen the herbalists' role as using plants to support the flow of that vital force. A classic example lies in the tendency of clinical herbalists and folk herbalists alike to see a fever as a healthy rallying of the vital force to drive out infection—a position that is increasingly shared by modern biomedicine. Rather than suppressing the fever with cooling herbs, herbalists tend to use herbs that release tension to relax the muscles and allow the blood to flow out to the periphery, so that it opens the pores, allowing the body to sweat and release excess heat.

What is anxiety but a psychic fever trying to move through a body that will not give it full expression? Yet most herbalists today try to subdue anxiety using large doses of herbs that dampen brain activity by the same mechanism—stimulation of the GABA receptors—as pharmaceutical anxiety medications. In my practice, I have found much better results by giving people herbs that release tension and encouraging them to let the anxiety move. Usually I begin cautiously, with a slow release of tension, to keep people from getting overwhelmed. Sometimes it is necessary to use some subtly cooling herbs to calm an overreactive nervous system, but here I prefer to use Rose family plants like Hawthorn (*Crataegus* spp.) that reduce hyperreactivity or small doses of bitter mints like Skullcap (*Scutellaria* spp.) that bring awareness down into the body by stimulating the enteric nervous system rather than large doses of GABAergic herbs like Valerian (*Valeriana* spp.). The bitter mints do tend to have GABAergic activity in higher doses, so I like to keep the dose low unless I am dealing with quieting the effects of physiological nerve pain. The GABA system is complex, and there are good reasons for engaging it directly, but doing it in a blunt force way is like icing an injury: it may bring some potential relief, but it will slow healing.

I learned the importance of that slow release several summers ago when I was beginning to get to know a few of the many species of the *Pedicularis* genus, plants with an amazing gift for relaxing muscular tension. When I am getting to know a plant, I often act like an awkward and overly enthusiastic teenager with a crush and end up trying to immerse myself in everything related to that plant.

So it was, that August, when I became infatuated with *Pedicularis*. I went into the mountains with a friend and found a beautiful streambed lined with *Pedicularis racemosa*—delicate plants with ethereal white flowers. For every three of the plants that I put into a mason jar for tincturing, I ate one or two. By late afternoon, my world was shimmering. Leaving the streambed, we found a stand of *Pedicularis groenlandica* dried out in the sun, and I decided to take some of that species home as well.

The next morning, I filled the bathtub with *Pedicularis groenlandica*, and while I soaked, I took a big dose of a *Pedicularis bracteosa* tincture someone had sent me. When I got out of the bath, I went to an acu-puncture session. I told the acupuncturist that I wanted to release ten-sion. So she needled Kidney 1 or KID 1, a point called *yongquan*, which means "bubbling spring."

Now, most people find the stimulation of Kidney 1 to be deeply grounding. What I did not know at the time, and what that acupunc-turist may or may not have known, is that the spring can bubble in different directions. Usually people feel the spring—the energy being moved—draining downward, carrying tension out through the bottom of their feet. But the spring can also bubble upward, stirring up the emotion that the tension has held in. That is what happened to me that day. After the appointment, I sobbed for six hours straight.

I was lucky in some ways, because I understood most of what hap-pened: I knew that as tension was releasing, emotion built up behind it. I was fine. Mostly. For better or worse, I tend to be someone who goes for big, cathartic releases. But I knew that not everyone would emerge from that kind of experience okay, especially if they did not have a framework for understanding what they were experiencing.

What kinds of plants release tension? Plants that engage the para-sympathetic. When we speak of anxiety, fear, anger, terror, and wild grief, we tend to speak of the activation of the sympathetic response—the fight-or-flight response. But what is actually happening is the dis-engagement of the parasympathetic response. In the absence of the connective instincts represented by the parasympathetic, the sym-pathetic tries to drive and focus us toward dealing with an external threat in an urgent and single-minded way. If we have faced similar threats before, we default to whatever response kept us from being killed in the past.

When we reengage the parasympathetic, we reorient ourselves in time and place. If we discover that we are actually safe, we become calm, and the nervous system begins finding another way to respond to the stimulus that triggered our fear. If this happens early enough in the process and is repeated frequently enough in similar situations, our brains will eventually reinterpret the meaning of the associated sensations in more benign terms. If we discover we are not actually safe in that moment but are able to regain a grounded, embodied presence through reengaging the parasympathetic, we will instinctively seek out more connective ways to resolve the situation—through negotiation or through seeking help from others.

There are three kinds of plants that I seek out in these situations. Each engages the parasympathetic slightly differently—acrid-tasting plants, bitter plants, and aromatic plants.

The swiftest and strongest parasympathetic reset comes from acrid-tasting plants. The acrid taste is a burning sensation experienced in the back of the throat at a point where the vagus nerve meets the tissues of the esophagus. Many plant and fungal alkaloids taste acrid. Some steroidal or triterpenoid saponins, including some cardiac glycosides, are acrid as well. Lobeline, an alkaloid found in the genus *Lobelia,* can be considered the archetypal acrid compound. The strong signal sent along the ventral branch of the vagus nerve awakens and connects all of our primary nerve centers—those in the pelvis, solar plexus, heart, and brain—instantly reorienting us. This reactivates the parasympathetic response and results in an immediate relaxation of tension: opening and deepening the breath, dilating the blood vessels, and bringing oxygenated blood, and hence awareness, back to areas cut off from circulation and sensation by constriction. This allows new signals to travel to and from all of our organs, except the adrenal medulla, the sole internal organ not innervated by nerves branching from the vagus and the organ whose influence becomes strongest when the vagal signal is at its weakest. Stimulate the acrid taste receptor too strongly, and you can make someone throw up. But sometimes that vomiting can be cathartic, helping a person have a visceral experience of releasing something poisonous that had entered her body.

Strongly bitter plants can have a similar effect through a different mechanism. All terpenes and all alkaloids have some degree of bitterness. The bitter taste is first experienced on the tongue, where a pair of cranial nerves carry it to the amygdala, which signals the liver and gall bladder to begin secreting bile, the stomach to release its digestive secretions, and the mouth to begin to salivate, all of which can only occur through parasympathetic engagement. This digestive stimulation also brings awareness down out of the head and into the solar plexus. Extremely bitter compounds—mostly alkaloids, but some terpenes as well—also have a strong action on the bitter taste receptors in the respiratory tract and the lower digestive tract and possibly in the heart, if they pass into the bloodstream in sufficient quantities. Very, very bitter plants like Gentian and Wormwood can bring about a strong reset response throughout the nervous system, much as acrid plants do. The extreme bitterness of the mescaline in San Pedro and Peyote cacti and the plants used to make Ayahuasca may be partially responsible for preparing the body to become more open to sensations as the brain becomes more open to new sensory input, allowing for a more dramatic kind of neurological reset, which we will talk more about soon. That extreme bitterness is definitely responsible for the cathartic vomiting those medicines can induce. In the Native American Church, when someone vomits during a ceremony, instead of saying that person got sick, they say that he got well. The Native American Church has a better track record of curing people of the poison of alcohol addiction than almost any other group.

Aromatic plants, those rich in the light terpenes and light phenols, which allow plants to communicate with each other through the air, are the gentlest relaxants. The olfactory nerve carries the news of their presence to the amygdala, which immediately recognizes it as the sign of the presence of our wild green kindred and activates the parasympathetic so we can receive the messages the plants are bringing.

Plants that engage the parasympathetic bring us back to ourselves and to each other, allowing healing to begin. From there, we can open more deeply to the wild and to the Otherworld as well, which give us new context for reimagining our lives.

They called Suibhne mad
because he preferred
the bugling of the Red Deer
to the sounds of the horn
and the hunt
and fled the company
of his fellow men
for a forest
then so vast
he could leap
from tree to tree.
One footstep
on his wild road
and you too
will find
madness,
or poetry,
or death.
The art lies
in resolving
madness
into poetry
to forestall death.
Dream enough
of the Roebuck
and the robeless king
and you will find yourself
wandering down
an bóthar fiáin,
not noticing
when the path

gives way to a Deer trail
and then the opening
created by the way
roots follow
underground streams
until you kneel down
among the Alders
at the water's edge,
digging Calamus
the fire of its root
lighting the fire at your root
and the fire in your heart
and the fire in your head
which spill forth
from your lips
as you join
in the song
of the Blackbirds
calling the world
to flower
and fruit
and seed
once more.

5
The Silver Branch

A few months after I turned nineteen, I ate the dried fruiting bodies of *Psilocybe* (*Psilocybe* spp.) mushrooms for the first time.

It was midautumn—the season when my Irish ancestors knew that the Otherworld was drawing near. Echoing the traditions of their prophet-poets (fili) in ways we did not know or understand at the time, a friend and I fasted for a day and then ate the mushrooms and wandered into the forest, seeking a new understanding of ourselves and our places in the world.

Walking up the trail, I felt my body begin to shift. I grew soft brown and white fur and then antlers, becoming a Stag. I began to nibble on twigs and evergreen leaves. I knew what it was to take the life of the forest into my body.

Then my attention shifted to the mosses growing on the granite hillside and the microcosm of the forest that I saw in its form when I got down to ground level.

Soon, my mind moved underground and felt the roots of the trees intertwining and filaments running between them, weaving together the mind of the forest, my own mind weaving together with it, remembering that I was made of earth and would return to earth, and that my life was not truly separate from any other life, my mind was not truly separate from any other mind. It was a deepening of a truth I had known innately since I was a young child wandering among the Maples and Oaks and Birches and Skunk Cabbage of the swamp behind my family's house.

It would be more than a decade before I would learn that the mushrooms I had eaten served the ecological role of creating the neural architecture of landforms and longer still until I would understand the connection between the world beneath our feet, the Otherworld of my ancestors, the shape-shifting that marks travel between those worlds, and the ways in which *Psilocybe* mushrooms can permanently transform our consciousness.

There is no reliable information about whether *Psilocybe* was part of the landscape of my Irish ancestors. I find it hard to believe, however, that it would not have been. Cattle were brought to Ireland and began to play a central role in Irish culture during the Neolithic, the same era when they began to build the great burial mounds now known as the sidhe—a word closely associated with the Otherworld English speakers call the Faerie realm and its denizens. Liberty Cap mushrooms (*Psilocybe semilanceata*) are abundant in the Irish countryside today, fruiting just before Samhain, the time of honoring the ancestors and the dead.

Psilocybe mushrooms play an integral role in the ecologies of grass-lands grazed by Bison, Sheep, Cattle, and other ungulates around the world. They enmesh themselves intimately with the roots of the grasses that shape their landscape. Stephen Buhner describes the process in detail:

> They, in essence, intertwine themselves with the root cellular tissues, penetrating the cells and cellular spaces. The specific zone of the root, where the plant and the fungal hyphae meet, is the cortex. The apex, or the part of the root considered to be the main neural structure, is not touched. A sheath or collar forms around the hyphae where it touches the living tissues of the root. This acts as a metabolic zone of interaction between the two where a constant exchange of chemical compounds occurs. The serotonergic

alkaloids in the fungal hyphae stimulate, as they do in all organisms, the development of new neurons, the formation of new neural networks, and the maturation of the cells of the plant root/brain system. Some of the outlying parts of the root system, already becoming senescent, experience an acceleration of that maturation, moving more quickly into senescence; that is, they get old and die. The *Psilocybe* then exists as a saprophytic organism, living on the decaying root mass. From this decaying root system, and from the living roots as well, the fungi gain nutrients and other compounds that aid their growth, particularly brassinosteroids, potent plant hormones. The fungal mycelium uses this compound, in essence, as a plant adaptogen, that is, a substance which enhances nonspecific resistance to environmental stressors. *Psilocybe* mushrooms are particularly fond of it.[1]

They are thus inextricably connected with the life, death, and consciousness of the plants with whom they form relationships. Together, the roots of the plants and the mycelia of the mushrooms form a fungal mat. Buhner continues:

> In healthy grasslands, over 1,000 species of vascular plants can also be found. And these vascular plants exist in a matrix formed by the psilocybe/grass endomycorrhizal mat which is in fact a three—dimensional topological space that extends from the depth of the deepest roots to the top of the highest tree in the range and from side-to-side, over the undulating landscape, as far as its boundaries flow. And this mat extends throughout the soil in that eco range. In essence, the ectomycorrhizal network—which is composed of a hybrid organism formed between plant neurons and fungal mycelial neurons at unique synaptic connections—forms an extensive neural system for that eco range. The other vascular plants form an integral part of this, for their root neurons are connected into the network as well.[2]

This mycorrhizal network is the physical structure that gives rise to the collective consciousness that is the mind of the land itself. The ecosystem experiences itself, on one level, as a single entity, responding to shared opportunities and shared threats. Our own nervous systems, and the consciousness that arises from them, are variations on this evolutionary theme—unifying the mind of the ecological communities we call bodies. The arising of a mycorrhizal network is an event in which a part of the world becomes locally self-aware. The formation of an individual nervous system is an event in which a part of an ecosystem develops another kind of local consciousness—but one that can only be healthy when woven into the web of connection it arises from.

Consciousness is shaped by the events within the synaptic networks that give rise to it and is reshaped by these events as well. A neural architecture takes on the shape of the gestalt of perceptions, sensations, and memories it carries, which becomes the shape of its map of the world. When its world changes, it must shift shape in order to navigate its changing reality.

This is where the shape-shifting neurotransmitters come in. Serotonin-like compounds like psilocybin serve to allow that network to take in a larger volume of sensory information by expanding their synaptic network and also to synthesize that information in new ways because the rapid branching these molecules stimulates occurs in a fractal way. This is true in every neural network they operate within. Buhner hypothesized that their evolutionary role was to help ecosystems develop novel responses to collective challenges. They serve this role for human brains too, in part by opening our awareness to the Otherworld.

John Moriarty would often say that this world and the Otherworld are part of the same Great World.[3] It is a way of seeing and being that until very recently was kept alive through unbroken traditions of thought and language going back to the Neolithic among native Irish speakers. In ancient Irish cosmology, the primary direction of passage to the Otherworld is downward: through a stone chamber or a cave or a deep lake, down to the well in the Otherworld where all our waters have their source. It is there that we can remember our own place of origin, remember our true nature. But to remember who we are is a perilous thing. It means we can never again allow ourselves to believe the small, narrow stories we have told ourselves about our entities in order to navigate our political, social, and economic lives.

There is no surviving Irish creation story, but some say that the ancient world was called forth from beneath the waters by the son of the sea, Mannanán mac Lir. That sea, like all the waters of the world, emerged from the Otherworld Well. Mannanán is a paradox—a god (we will complicate that word in a bit) of misty waters who is honored on the brightest day of the year, a wild god whose rage is the storm who is also the source of the most sublime music of enchantment, a sea god who cannot see water as we do, but instead sees the ocean as a field of wildflowers. He is a protector of the innocent and a consoler of the grieving who also has a laugh that echoes off the mountains and water and fills the sky and the lustiness of the wild white horses that are the crashing waves of the cold North Atlantic.

The departure of the Tuath Dé, the Tribe of the Gods, from the world of the living and their transformation into the Daoine Sidhe was achieved through Mannanán's magic—magic of revelation and disappearance, magic of mists and of clear vision.

The Tuath Dé had come to Ireland early in the history of the world, sailing on ships carried through the sky by the north wind to wage a war to free the island from the brutal rule of Balor, a wicked king who demanded human sacrifice and whose single-eyed gaze corrupted and withered all it looked upon. In many ways, we can see him as the personification and embodiment of the spirit that would become first civilization and then empire and then colonialism and then global capitalism, overrunning the world. Mannanán was already there when the Tuath Dé arrived. He was one of the older, wilder gods who became their kin and their teacher. He trained his foster son, Lugh, in the martial and magical arts, and Lugh blinded and slew Balor with a single thrust of a spear made of sunlight.

In time, though, new invaders came, Galatian Celts from Spain. Modern scholars verify that Celtic people arrived in Ireland from Spain in the Bronze Age and that another people existed there before them. (Interestingly, long ago, when the first Oak trees were growing in Europe, Ireland and Spain were part of the same landmass, and their oldest trees are genetically related.)

In that time, Mannanán had become one of the kings of the Tuath Dé, even though he had not been born among them, and he sought to drive back the invaders by calling up a storm. But the bard of the Galatians, Amergin, seduced the land and the sea with a song that calmed the storm, and then, standing on the hill of Uisneach as the Hawthorn bloomed, called forth a new world that supplanted the old one. Magan writes that "Amergin became a leader of the island, and his first act was to begin uttering an incantation, summoning up the world that he intended to create here and clarifying the interrelation between it and all the other planes of existence, physical and spiritual."[4] That new world was a harsher place than the one that came before it, and it has no place for the Tuath Dé, whose ways, as Victor Anderson said, were "kinder and less civilized."

So, Mannanán gathered his people under a mound at the mouth of the Bóinne, the river that mirrors the Milky Way, and showed them another world below, the world from which all things in this world emerge, the world to which the dead return. He divided among them the Hollow Hills that were the common tombs of the Neolithic people of Ireland and showed them how to pass into the Otherworld from this world through those tombs. When they made that passage, the Tuath Dé became the Daoine Sidhe, the People of the Mound.

He also taught them an incantation, Mannanán's Cloak, that allowed them to remain shrouded from human sight when they pass into this world. But like all things of wind and water and word, the conjured cloak is a fleeting thing, and like all cloaks sometimes it slips. So our new world defends itself against incursions from the Otherworld through its own incantations, asserting our separation from the rest of life, which remains and moves freely through both worlds, and armoring ourselves against its life-changing insights through constantly reasserting an ideology that, with repetition, reshapes our neural networks and blocks out information that might force their expansion. The serotonergic compounds we call psychedelic lift both veils and open passageways—for good or for ill.

Since childhood, I have felt that when the Tuath Dé left this realm, they took with them ways of knowing and being essential to the wholeness of the world. I always wanted to travel to the Otherworld—sometimes to dwell there, sometimes to bring what was taken there back into this world. When I ate the fruiting bodies of the mushrooms whose mycelial tendrils weave into the world, at a half-conscious level, this is what I sought. Though I did not know his name, through the mushrooms, I was calling on Mannanán.

Mannanán was not and is not without mercy for those of this world who would truly honor the ways of his people. From time to time, he has come into this world bearing a silver branch bedecked with golden Apples from the Otherworld. Who holds the branch can see the world as he does, the world refracted through the teardrop of his Beloved's beauty. The great ancient Irish king Cormac mac Art (Cormac Son of the Bear) heard heavenly music when Mannanán shook the branch. When Cormac himself held it, he beheld the Otherworld Well wherein the Salmon of Wisdom dwells.

The encounter with Mannanán is a powerful initiation. Moriarty writes:

Never are we so challenged in all that we are as when we encounter Mannanán.

The instant we meet him we know that eye and mind are habits of eye and mind.

The instant we meet him we know that the world we have lived in was all along but a habit of seeing, a habit of knowing.

The instant we meet him we know that being human is a habit, and, walking away, we know how shaken in that habit we now are.[5]

This is a shift to experiencing the world as "gods" do. (I promised we would come back to this word.)

Victor Anderson told Cornelia Benavidez that his tradition, the Feri tradition, "is a nature way, it's the way of Nature, and it's a way of accepting and developing all your talents, all of your nature in such a way that you are worthy to be called a god in the making." This mirrors some interesting understandings in old Irish tradition. Some of the oldest Irish texts contain a curious phrase: *dée ocus andée*, meaning "god and not-gods." Analyzing these texts, Celtic Reconstructionist scholar Annie Loughlin writes:

> The *Cóir Anmann* attempts to explain the meaning by saying that "*Dée* were the poets and *an-dée* the husbandmen," and "These were their gods, the magicians, and their non-gods were husbandmen." The *Lebor Gabála Érenn* follows suit. Of the Tuatha Dé Danann, then, we are led to believe that there were those who were skilled in the arts (*dé*), and those who were not (*andé*), but were still of the same race, the same people. Effectively, it is the skill (and resulting status) of the *dé* that set them apart from their fellow people and marks out their divine status. That certainly fits with what myths like *Cath Maige Tuired* tells us about the Tuatha Dé being skilled in the arts, for one—that they "were in the northern islands of the world, studying occult lore and sorcery, druidic arts and witchcraft and magical skill, until they surpassed the sages of the Pagan arts."[6]

What were the arts that the gods perfected? Drawing from the work of Tomás Ó Rathile (Anglicized as Thomas O'Rahilly), a great Irish scholar who was instrumental in the early twentieth-century movement to revitalize the Irish language, Anthony Murphy writes:

> O'Rahilly tells us that some characteristics of an "Otherworld deity" such as Dagda were his omniscience (rofhessa, "great knowledge") and his polymorphism. The Otherworld deity was regularly considered to

possess the ability to assume an animal shape, for example a bull, a wolf, a pig, a hawk, an eagle or a swan. However, when the Otherworld was located beneath the sea or a lake or body of water, it would take the "appropriate" shape for a "denizen of the waters"—a salmon.[7]

As such, the Salmon of Wisdom might well be understood as the part of a god that has delved the world's greatest depths. Shape-shifting is a fundamental attribute of gods and a necessary skill for a god in the making to acquire.

This is further supported by the sense given by many old Irish stories that reincarnation and the memory of different forms a person had inhabited was not something every soul accomplished, but rather an ordeal great souls moved through in the process of becoming heroes or chieftains or magicians or queens or kings. This could occur through the grace of encountering a magical being who you treated with great respect—or as a punishment for treating a denizen of the Otherworld with disrespect. Robin Artisson writes:

When we study the ancient notion of the many souls as displayed in the Fayerie tales or ballads, we come into contact with very old pre-Christian cultural material. The soul (or the many souls) are depicted as able to transform into birds, plants, animals, and many other shapes. The reality of shape-shifting is ubiquitous for spirits and Otherworldly entities and for many parts of the human soul-complex. This reveals the soul's natural kinship to the Unseen world and its primal inherence within that extraordinary realm. And this reveals the necessarily relational nature of the many souls. To shape-shift implies altering and transformative influences coming to bear on the person or their souls, through various sorts of relationships. These can be friendly influences endowing a man or woman's souls with shape-shifting power aligned with their will, or they can be hostile, transforming them against their will. These influences can also be purely neutral, like the natural processes of aging or death that bring about transformations in various degrees in all entities subject to them.[8]

There is a striking similarity between this kind of experience and the experiences the rogue psychologist and psychedelic pioneer Timothy Leary associated with the activation of certain levels of consciousness. While imprisoned in the 1970s, through correspondence and conversation with his friend Robert Anton Wilson and his wife at the time, Joanna Harcourt-Smith, Leary developed a model of eight circuits of consciousness. The awakening of each circuit of consciousness, according to the model, involves rearranging the cognitive map of the world based on becoming reoriented and reimprinted to another level of outward reality, beginning with the orientation to our original source of nourishment. The nature of our relationship with the external reality that shapes our imprint shapes the neural architecture we create during that phase and the sense of self that emerges from it—the habits of being and perception we adopt, to retranslate it into Moriarty's terms.

The first four circuits develop organically in most people as they mature toward adulthood: first-circuit concerns revolve around seeking nourishment and physical safety; second-circuit concerns revolve around questions of territory; third-circuit concerns involve creating a fixed mental map of reality, which functional magnetic resonance imaging (fMRI) studies suggest may be a function of the parahippocampus;[9] and fourth-circuit concerns revolve around sexuality. The "higher" circuits correspond to functions connected with what our culture defines as the spiritual realm.

The activation of the fifth circuit results in understanding the provisional nature of our maps of reality as a precursor to understanding other "worlds." The sixth-circuit activation involves releasing and rewriting our social relationships and identities. Recent fMRI research suggests that this can occur in psychedelic states due to a change in the relationship between the parahippocampus, which is responsible for the creation and maintenance of aspects of memory involving the "spatial configurations of objects but not object identity, and that this takes place independent of the hippocampus,"[10] and the retro splenial cortex, which may help to situate us in space: "decreased connectivity between the parahippocampus and retro splenial cortex (RSC) correlated strongly with ratings of 'ego-dissolution' and 'altered meaning,' implying the importance of this particular circuit for the maintenance of 'self' or 'ego' and its processing of 'meaning.'"[11]

This may partially explain why *Psilocybe* mushrooms are sometimes effective in treating trauma, which involves deep identification with past experiences that reshape our experience of ourselves, and depression, which is often rooted in our understanding of our relationship to the world around us. People who have good results in using *Psilocybe* mushrooms to treat depression show decreased connectivity between the parahippocampus and the prefrontal cortex, as well as decreased activation of the amygdala, which, among other things, is involved in our fear responses, several weeks after treatment.[12]

This opens the way for seventh-circuit experiences—which are essentially experiences of shape-shifting, reincarnation, and direct experience of the union of all things. Modern psychedelic researchers refer to these as experiences of "oceanic boundlessness." Leary, Wilson, and Harcourt-Smith described the eighth circuit as the capacity to alter the structure of time and space—but they admitted that they had not yet encountered anyone who had activated the eighth circuit and come back to tell the tale.

Leary and Wilson described in an essay the seventh-circuit reality.

The seventh brain kicks into action when the nervous system begins to receive signals from *within the individual neuron*, from the DNA-RNA dialogue. The first to achieve this mutation spoke of "memories of past lives," "reincarnation," "immortality," etc. That these adepts were recording something real is indicated by the fact that many of them (especially Hindus and Sufis) gave marvelously accurate poetic vistas of evolution 1,000 or 2,000 years before Darwin and foresaw Superhumanity before Nietzsche. The "akashic records" of Theosophy, the "collective unconscious" of Jung, the "phylogenetic unconscious" of Groff and Ring, are three modern metaphors for this circuit. These visions of past and future evolution described by those who have had "out-of-body" experiences during close-to-death episodes also describe circuit VII tunnel-reality. . . . The [primary] specific circuit VII neurotransmitter is, of course, LSD. (Peyote and psilocybin can produce some circuit VII experiences also.) Circuit VII is best considered, in terms of 1977 science, as the genetic archives, activated by anti-histone proteins. [It is worth noting that Leary and Wilson wrote these words before the role of histamine in creating aversive memory had been established.] The DNA memory coiling back to the dawn of life. A sense of the inevitability of immortality and interspecies symbiosis comes to all circuit VII mutants.[13]

These experiences involve imprinting on the world itself—transcending individuated reality and then artfully returning to one's own body. I believe this accounts for some of the success people have in working with *Psilocybe* mushrooms to resolve fear, depression, and anxiety at the end of life. It calls to mind my experience of giving these mushrooms to a man who had recently received a cancer diagnosis. As we walked together through the woods, he saw how his molecules would be recycled into the body of the world and he too could become part of the forest and how the imprint of his being would live on in the ways he had changed the lives of everyone he knew. His sense of self expanded and shifted in a way that allowed him to understand that we are all, essentially, shape-shifting immortals.

There are perils we can encounter when shape-shifting our sense of selfhood. One set of dangers involves setting out without proper intention or conducting ourselves in an untoward manner and ending up in a dangerous place. Not everything that dwells in this realm or in other realms is friendly toward us, and when we act in rash or foolish or disrespectful ways, we stand a greater chance of encountering the hostile sides of dangerous beings. In the vulnerable and malleable state the medicine of *Psilocybe* puts us in, this can result in our taking on a dangerous imprint. Traditionally, this was referred to as possession. It has its correlate in modern understandings of brainwashing.

Timothy Leary described the ways in which Charles Manson warped the psyches of his followers by using Benzedrine and LSD in combination with techniques developed by magical adepts: "Manson used drugs as but one brainwashing tool, and he did so for ends alien to the drug culture. While other gurus of the sixties used drugs to rewire their followers for the peace-love-ecology trip, Manson used the same drugs to imprint his family for fascism, racism, sexism."[14] Leary was aware that his own government had experimented with LSD as a way to control human behavior.

By immersing his followers in an environment he controlled, and then using LSD to make their nervous systems malleable, Manson created a situation in which they imprinted not on the collective mind of the living world, but on Manson himself and the cult he was building. Leary went on to say: "Brainwashing, like malaria, is a disease of exposure. Put people in a malarial environment and most of them will get malaria. Put them in a brainwashing institution and most of them will get brainwashed."[15]

I will admit that while I welcome the beginning of the relaxation of laws against psychedelics, I worry a great deal about the ways in which corporations, medical institutions, and religious groups will engineer experiences of these medicines that, while not overt attempts at brain-washing, will leave people vulnerable to imprinting on the consciousness of a human institution. To be certain, few if any psychedelic researchers are interested in brainwashing people, and for all its flaws, our medical system does not consciously seek to manipulate people. But that does not mean that a clinical setting and a clinical mind-set will not shape people's experiences in very particular ways.

Most people in this culture take the clinical nature of medicine as a given, but as French philosopher and cultural historian Michel Foucault documented in *The Birth of the Clinic*, it is an approach to healing that had its origins in the seventeenth century—concurrent with the rise of the mechanistic worldview and the emergence of capitalism. The clinic as setting is a sterile space, intended to create a neutral atmosphere. But there is no such thing as true neutrality. Attempts at neutrality actually result in erasing context and stripping an experience of the meaning that context gives. And the sterility of the clinic gives rise to a particular mind-set that both shapes and is shaped by that physical setting—this is no less true if the harshness of bright lights, white walls, and cold metal are replaced by softer lighting, softer furniture, and softer colors. Foucault writes: "The clinic—constantly praised for its empiricism, the modesty of its attention, and the care with which it silently lets things surface to the observing gaze without disturbing them with discourse—owes its real importance to the fact that it is a reorganization in depth, not only of medical discourse, but of the very possibility of a discourse about disease."[16] That medical gaze that Foucault speaks of seeks to objectify both the patient and the patient's experience. The discourse of disease that it gives rise to is one that views the body as a discrete, self-contained machine that breaks down in particular predictable ways that can be corrected according to certain set protocols.

Psychedelics in general and psilocybin in particular don't really operate in ways that fit this approach. The nature of a fungal organism is to make connections, to weave together ecologies, and to create complex information networks that give rise to novel perceptions and solutions.

Many contemporary researchers and advocates of psychedelic medicine espouse the narrative that the counterculture of the 1960s gave psychedelics a bad name and that we need to eschew its insights and approaches in favor of clinical discourse and medical legitimacy. They seek to tame the medicines. Pharmacologist Roland Griffiths, considered by many to be the researcher who ushered in the current psychedelic renaissance, told *Scientific American* that he felt psilocybin was best administered in a clinical context "like an anesthetic being dispensed and managed by an anesthesiologist"—a carefully controlled experience designed to produce a predictable result.[17]

Paradoxically, Griffiths and most of his colleagues recognize the importance of the mystical and spiritual aspects of the psychedelic

experience. Studies of the effectiveness of psilocybin in the ameliora-
tion of the fear of death in patients with terminal diagnoses, depression, and addiction repeatedly show that the best predictor of success
is a person's openness to the experience of oceanic boundlessness. But
they miss the irony of creating a tightly bound context for inviting
people into that experience of boundlessness.

The conditions that these clinicians seek to treat emerge from a cri-
sis of meaning. Trauma and the addictions that result from it are connected with deep identification with particular events and situations in
the past that ossify the structure and perception of the self. Depression
is a loss of connection to the world we live in. The anxiety connected
with facing death is tied in with the idea that we are finite, discrete
beings and that when we as individuals die we cease to exist. Foucault
saw this view of death as a product of the clinical mind-set. He said that
with the rise of modern medicine, "Death left its old tragic heaven and
became the lyrical core of man: his invisible truth, his visible secret"[18]—
the secret that shapes identity and experience.

The same is true of the softer version of the clinical approach to
psychedelics, the "wellness" approach. Last year, Jonah Bromwich of
the *New York Times* reported that many of the same investment firms
that have been driving the rise of companies like Goop and Moon
Juice, which market high-end products and treatments to discontented
wealthy people, are seeking to expand the wellness industry to include
companies marketing psychedelics. Describing the philosophy of one
of the venture capital funds investing in Compass's psilocybin research
and development, Bromwich writes: "This year, Able has publicly dedicated itself to narrowing what its partners call 'the wellness gap.' That's
how they describe the distance between standard economic measures of
prosperity and how rotten everyone feels all the time."[19]

In the context of this vision, a psilocybin treatment becomes a way
to achieve relief from ennui—but, again, without addressing the roots
of that ennui. To do so would mean challenging the ideological framework that creates the wealth-generating economic structures that enable

customers to pay for these experiences, undermining the lifestyle the wellness movement wants to promote.

The power of psilocybin lies in its ability to change our relationships with ourselves and the world. This happens when we engage the medicine on its own terms—embracing the unpredictability of the experience and seeking not just to relieve symptoms or eliminate undesirable traits, but also to truly connect with something outside and beyond our existing frameworks of understanding. The degree to which someone is ready to have their understanding of the world transformed and let go of their stories of who they are marks the degree to which a person will gain wisdom and insight from working with mushrooms The openness to the experience of one's own infinity seems to be the primary predictor of success when *Psilocybe* mushrooms are used to treat depression:

> In line with previous reports, we hypothesized that the occurrence and magnitude of Oceanic Boundlessness (OBN) (sharing features with mystical-type experience) and Dread of Ego Dissolution (DED) (similar to anxiety) would predict long-term positive outcomes. . . .
>
> To summarize, the occurrence of high OBN (sharing features with mystical-type experience) and low DED (relating to anxiety and impaired cognition) under psilocybin predicted positive clinical outcomes in a trial of psilocybin for TRD [treatment-resistant depression]. This relationship exhibited a degree of specificity, in that psilocybin-induced OBN was significantly more predictive of reduced depressive symptoms than the drug's more generic visual and auditory perceptual effects.[20]

This shift in identification also results in a shift in our experience of empathy, which puts us at odds with the dominant culture, creating a third danger of social and cultural exile. But many who take up the path of the Silver Branch have already felt like exiles their entire lives.

In our culture, ideology places strong limits on our ability to empathize with plants, animals, fungi, mountains, and rivers. Most Christians believe that their god created other-than-human life for the benefit of humans and gave reason to humans alone. Secular capitalism removes God from the equation but retains Christianity's view that other forms of life exist for our benefit. Contemporary progressive ideologies, from "woke" capitalism to the blend of identity politics and socialism that passes for left-ist discourse in America today, do acknowledge the importance of plants, animals, and places that are sacred to Indigenous cultures, but their value is still predicated on their relationship to particular groups of humans, a valuation that ultimately fails to take seriously the underpinnings and implications of the animist worldviews of the cultures people claim to be protecting. These same ideologies tend to be suspicious of those who defend wild creatures and wild places outside the context of Indigenous struggles, treating compassion and concern as limited resources that must be redistributed in ways that balance patterns of human injustice, often implying that one cannot simultaneously care deeply about mercury in the blood of Loons and lead in the blood of children.

This is not inherent to the human condition. Throughout most of the history of our species, most humans have experienced plants, ani-mals, and fungi as conscious beings and as members of their extended communities to whom they owe compassion and respect. Many cultures speak of these beings as our elder relatives or our brother and sister rela-tives. This reflects an instinctual and intuitive knowledge of the ori-gins of our consciousness. Consciousness is widely distributed in nature. Our current biological model of consciousness recognizes it as an emer-gent phenomenon of complex living systems on scales ranging from communities of bacteria to individual multicellular organisms to the local mycorrhizal networks of ecosystems to entire planets. Our neural networks are variations on the rhizomes of plants and the mycelia of fungi. The neurotransmitters that regulate signaling across these net-works are a molecular inheritance from ancient bacteria. They are the very same compounds that promote the growth of and regulate signal-ing across the mycorrhizal networks that form the biological structure of the minds of forests and fields.[21]

So it should come as no surprise that the compounds of plants and fungi that are most closely related to the neurotransmitter that allows us to feel what other beings are feeling, serotonin, have the capacity to increase our capacity to feel empathy for and connection with other-than-human life. In a study of people who had belief-changing experiences while working with Ayahuasca, *Psilocybe* spp. mushrooms, LSD (a semisynthetic derivative of the *Claviceps purpurea* fungus), DMT, and 5-MeO-DMT (natural or semisynthetic derivatives of a variety of plants and animals), all classic serotonergic psychedelics, researchers found that:

> From before the experience to after, there were large increases in attribution of consciousness to various entities including non-human primates (63–83%), quadrupeds (59–79%), insects (33–57%), fungi (21–56%), plants (26–61%), inanimate natural objects (8–26%), and inanimate manmade objects (3–15%). Higher ratings of mystical experience were associated with greater increases in the attribution of consciousness. Moreover, the increased attributions of consciousness did not decrease in those who completed the survey years after the psychedelic experience. In contrast to attributions of consciousness, beliefs in freewill and superstitions did not change. Notably, all findings were similar when restricted to individuals reporting on their first psychedelic experience.[22]

This is supported by an earlier finding that patients being given psilocybin to mitigate treatment-resistant depression experienced "increased nature relatedness."[23]

Such medicines change belief by taking us outside the structure of belief, expanding the sensory and emotional information available to us in ways that our previous fixed stories of the world cannot contain. Rigid belief is an odd fixation of our modern culture, one that arose in its current form with the institutionalization of Christianity and the formalization of its creed. For most of human history, lived, embodied experiences of encountering the living world and fluid cultural memory that lived through stories and songs created a more fluid mind-set less likely to confuse the map for the terrain. People did not "believe" or "disbelieve" in listening to the teachings of an Oak, conversing with Blackbirds, or receiving a message in a dream from the spirit of the river—they simply engaged in these experiences and made meaning from them in the context of their own experiences and the experiences of the members of their communities, living and dead. Ritual use of psychedelic medicines, together with music and dance and spontaneous poetic expression prevented ideas about the world from becoming too ossified. They can do the same for us now, when engaged in the right way.

The ability of these medicines to increase empathy for other-than-human life is rooted in the neurobiology of our oldest form of empathy, that which reflects the modern word's etymology, the ability to "feel with" other beings, a capacity that does not honor the limits ideology places on our compassion. It is also, not incidentally, related to their role in facilitating communication and promoting creativity in ecosystems when released by the fungi and plants that have been producing, releasing, and ingesting these compounds for far, far longer than humans have been on this planet.

Contemporary neurobiology understands empathy as coming in two forms, which balance each other: cognitive empathy, which involves correctly surmising the thoughts, emotions, and wishes of others based on facial expressions and verbal cues, and emotional or affective empathy, which involves sensory and emotional responses to other people's feelings. Our culture tends to favor cognitive empathy over emotional empathy.

As its name suggests, cognitive empathy involves the cognitive process of forming a hypothesis about someone else's mental state based on observations and past experiences. It is a function of the part of our being that operates in realms of abstraction. It really has very little to do with "feeling with" other beings at all. As such, it is closely associated with a person's "theory of mind," their understanding of how most humans perceived the world. Those whose cognitive empathy is considered strong by conventional assessments tend to have a model of others' mental and emotional states that tracks with the cognitive processes of the majority of humans. Conventional assessments of cognitive empathy do not take into account the ability to correctly assess the feelings, wants, and needs of neurodivergent people, because neurodivergent expressions of emotion are considered aberrant. Nor do they take into account the ability to correctly assess the feelings, wants, and needs of other-than-human beings. As such, cognitive empathy will always appear high in neurotypical people and also psychopaths. The latter, with high cognitive empathy and low emotional empathy, can easily manipulate people because we can accurately perceive the workings of others' minds but cannot feel their suffering. Because tests designed to measure cognitive empathy are based on the ability to correctly guess neurotypical people's thoughts and emotions based on their speech and facial expressions, Autistic people are conventionally seen as lacking in cognitive empathy. However, there is some evidence that Autistic people are better at reading Autistic facial expressions and verbal cues than neurotypical people are. We also tend to be better at reading neurotypical people's nonverbal cues than neurotypical people are at reading ours, because, as a survival skill we have had to learn to adapt to a world shaped by the neuromajority.

An aspect of cognitive empathy that I have not seen addressed elsewhere is that cognitive empathy, as a cognitive process, is influenced deeply by ideology. Our beliefs shape not only our interpretation of others' experiences, but our assessment of whose experiences are worth interpreting. Here I look to the work of the Italian Marxist philosopher Antonio Gramsci, who died in one of Mussolini's prisons in no small part because of his tendency to empathize with the "wrong" people. As Valeriano Ramos Jr. wrote, Gramsci "describ[ed] ideology as a 'terrain' of practices, principles, and dogmas having a material and institutional nature constituting individual subjects once these were 'inserted' into such a terrain . . . ideology constituted individuals as subjects and social agents in society."[24] Thus, ideology defines who is and who is not a person and whose experiences are worthy of our attention. Corporations, states, armies, and gangs maintain internal cohesiveness by defining their members as people worthy of care while defining their targets as less than human. Anthropocentric cultures engage in a similar process of limiting personhood to humans. Animist cultures recognize the personhood of all beings and thus consider all beings worthy of empathy.

Emotional empathy, being rooted in feeling rather than in abstraction, is less shaped by ideology. In some ways, I find emotional empathy to be a misleading term because in this culture, which has dissociated the mind from the body, we have a tendency to treat emotions as inconveniently irrational valences of thought. In reality, emotions are a kind of sensory information rather like an electromagnetic form of the sense of touch.[25] Just as touch is experienced by the sensory nerves along our skin and scent and taste are variations on touch, experienced by specialized epithelial tissues sensitive to the presence of certain kinds of molecules, emotion is an experience felt throughout the entire body in response to our nervous system's experiences of the presence of living beings—including our own presence and the presences conjured by our memories and our imaginations. So, in many ways, emotional memory might be better called somatic empathy. As such, it is a wilder form of empathy, one more rooted in our animal selves. It is, to quote a phrase Victor Anderson used to describe the Faerie realm, "kinder and less civilized." And our stories of the banishing of the denizens of that realm from this world to the Otherworld is, on one level, a story of our attempting to cage and tame emotional empathy.

As I write in *Courting the Wild Queen*, from the standpoint of our civilization:

> The trouble with such empathy is that it refuses to honor the rules of etiquette that guide civilization's preferred form of cognitive empathy, which is marked and tested by the ability to correctly guess the internal experience and the desired response of another person by thinking about the situation and running it through the rubric of the normative experiences and responses of the majority population. More subversively, this wild type of empathy refuses to honor the rules set for whom or what we may empathize with and whose experiences should

matter to us most. You are supposed to care more about the wellbeing of your family members than about the wellbeing of the man sleeping in the doorway of the bank, more about the death of an American soldier in a helicopter crash than about the deaths of twenty Yemeni civilians in a drone strike on a wedding party. And you are not supposed to empathize at all with trees or stones or rivers or stars. All those rules and categories break down when we bypass abstraction and go to a place of directly experiencing the presence of other beings.[26]

There are strong indications that emotional empathy is related to the neurotransmitter serotonin, part of our inheritance from ancient bacteria, which tended to operate as collectives. Psilocybin, produced by mushrooms of the *Psilocybe* genus, and LSD, related to compounds from the ergot fungus, are chemically similar to serotonin. The fungal realm is a realm of beings whose mode of consciousness is marked by connection and by curiosity—branching out in new directions in response to sensory stimuli, seeking to experience the world by embedding its structures of consciousness in soil, rock, and the bodies of other living and once-living things.[27]

Serotonin, psilocybin, and their molecular kin are compounds that facilitate the flow of sensory information across structures of consciousness and encourage the fractal branching of those networks to facilitate new ways of making connections. As such, they are molecules of embodied connection—molecules of empathy.

The relationship between serotonin and emotional empathy shows up in research into the chemical compound MDMA, dubbed an "empathogen" by the intrepid psychonaut and psychotherapist Ralph Metzner. MDMA is chemically similar to the neurotransmitter phenylethylamine, which, among other things, acts strongly on serotonin and dopamine receptors in a way similar to those two neurotransmitters themselves and to mescaline, the primary psychedelic alkaloid in Peyote (*Lophophora williamsii*), San Pedro (*Trichocereus pachanoi*), and Peruvian Torch (*Echinopsis peruviana*) cacti. One study, by Gilinder Bedi, David Hyman, and Harriet de Wit, found that "MDMA increased 'empathogenic' feelings, but it reduced accurate identification of threat-related facial emotional signals in others"[28]—a finding that would be consistent with an increase in emotional empathy and a decrease in cognitive empathy, though these researchers didn't make that connection. A pair of Bedi's colleagues, Lawrence Scahill and George Anderson, did, however, reach this conclusion, observing that "on balance, the findings presented in the Bedi et al. study indicate that although MDMA might enhance the emotional component of empathy, it appears to cause impairment in cognitive component."[29] All of the aforementioned researchers attribute the increase in emotional empathy brought on by MDMA at least in part to serotonin. A 2019 paper found that the tendency to increase feelings of empathy associated with MDMA is also shared by LSD and thus most likely by psilocybin.[30]

Those who find relief from depression with psilocybin report both a decreased tendency toward authoritarian attitudes and an increased affinity for nature.[31] This suggests a loosening of rigid belief structures and a possible increase in emotional empathy for other-than-human life. I would posit that these are both essential elements of the kind of belief-changing psychedelic experiences that researchers Sandeep Nayak and Roland Griffiths associate with an increased willingness to view plants and animals as conscious beings.[32] Viewing other beings as conscious is a necessary prerequisite to showing them compassion and respect.

An additional link between serotonin and empathy for other-than-human beings is also worth noting. Autistic people tend to have elevated levels of serotonin and to have weak cognitive empathy (at least compared to the internal experiences of neurotypical people) but strong emotional empathy.[33] Autistic people also often tend to have strong affinities for and identification with plants, animals, and other entities not typically treated as people within the dominant culture. Ralph Savarese, a literary scholar who has studied writing by a wide range of both speaking and nonspeaking Autistic people, notes that many Autistic narratives reflect deep empathy for beings and objects not commonly considered to possess subjectivity in the same way society assumes that humans do. He attributes this to the strong emotional empathy of Autistic people, which I, in turn, associate with elevated serotonin levels, which make the day-to-day experience of Autistic people rather psychedelic at times.[34]

Long periods of time in the wilderness also seem to elevate serotonin levels, in ways that tend to make one experience the world much like that of an Autistic person. Elevated levels of serotonin or serotonergic alkaloids are likely necessary factors in bringing about ecological empathy in someone raised in a nonanimist culture, but they are not likely to be sufficient. When a mind is being repatterned, what that mind is focused on is essential.

It is no small miracle that people receiving psilocybin treatment in clinical settings have still experienced an increase in "nature connectedness." How much more connected would these people have felt to the living world if they had been given their medicine in a forest instead of in a clinic? How much more connected would they have felt if, instead of being told they were given a pharmacological substance to treat their depression, they were told they were taking in the fruiting body of a living being that arose as an expression of the mind of a field in order to help them overcome their sense of isolation? And how much more connection yet would they have experienced the life cycle of those mushrooms?

The great gifts of such a medicine can only truly be received when accompanied by an invitation to understand that they are elder kin who we are meeting with to remember who we are, to be reminded of the nature of our consciousness.

Consciousness is the fruiting body of a vast mycelial organism whose tendrils entwine with the roots of ancient trees and ephemeral wildflowers. Songs and poems are spores on the wind, carrying all we have known and felt and been to new soil where life might begin its wild fractal branching again. We are part of Earth become individually conscious. We can heal ourselves by weaving back into the living web of consciousness from which we evolved and emerged. The medicines of connection and communication play an essential role in that reweaving.

We are water and stone and lightning and starlight that has danced through a thousand forms. Biology emerged from infinity so that the world could experience itself. Our individual neural networks evolved from mycorrhizal networks of consciousness that the world might view itself from outside itself and discover itself anew. Our languages follow patterns derived from the syntax of fungal communication—but carried through the air as sound vibrations, the traces of which we symbolically represent in writing. When we remember to embody the curiosity we evolved to experience, we remember, in the words of the Zen poet Dōgen, that the beings surround us are "others none other than ourselves."[35] If I have faith in anything, it is that such curiosity is our nature, and that in the presence of curiosity, cruelty becomes impossible. The ability of the psychedelic compounds produced by our plant and fungal kin to enhance that curiosity makes them potent allies in the revival of animism. The next step after working with these medicines to shift our perceptions is to reshape our lives in ways that root us in the world that we now truly know to be alive.

> The magic power of a poem consists in it always being filled with duende, in its baptising all who gaze at it with dark water.
>
> FEDERICO GARCÍA LORCA,
> "THEORY AND PLAY OF THE DUENDE"

> *Mad, dead, or a poet*
> *was never really*
> *a choice:*
> *once you have held*
> *the Silver Branch*
> *and gazed*
> *into the abyss*
> *that lies beneath*
> *the dark waters*

of the well
that feeds
the rivers
of the senses
and the rivers
of the world
you will
always
carry the
scent of the
Otherworld,
the obsidian
shimmer
of duende's
baptism
in dark water,
only poetry
can resolve
the torrents
of madness
into clarity,
only poetry
can shape
the breath
to feed
the fire
that feeds
the forge
of the heart
that shapes
the spirit
like the molten
iron

that rises up
from the
heart
of the earth
and sets
ablaze
the fire
at your root
and the fire
in your blood
and the fire
in your head
that blazes
in eyes
that shine
like the
Midsummer
bonefire
and pours
forth from
the tongue
in words
that
bless
and words
that curse
and words
that command
roots
to break
through
sidewalks
and forests

to rise
where cities
now stand,
that like
the wind
in the desert
Ezekiel knew
commands
the dry bones
to live.
The fires
of a burning
world
have leapt
into my head,
and find
their match
in the
scarlet leaves
reflected
in the water
and the
red light
of Mars
in the sky.
In times
like this
my ancestors
donned feather cloaks
and went alone
into the forest
and ate autumn's
strange Underworld fruit

*that bloomed forth
after the rains,
spread across
the ground
like Hazelnuts,
holding
the memory
the forest
infused
into the topsoil,
and gazed
into the waters
until the fire
cooled enough
for the visions
to condense
and rain down
as words
sweet enough
upon the tongue
to soothe
the way
truth burns,
and returned
to the people
hoping to conjure
in their hearts
the rhythm
and in their breath
the song
that would
make the
wasteland bloom.*

6
Rooting in the Living World

Stripped of our illusions, transformed by our bodies' experiencing the fertile life of the land, we can no longer continue to live in the ways of a culture that denies that the world is alive. Stephen Buhner writes of this:

> If we eat the wild, it begins to work inside us, altering us, changing us. Soon, if we eat too much, we will no longer fit the suit that has been made for us. Our hair will begin to grow long and ragged. Our gait and how we hold our body will change. A wild light begins to gleam in our eyes. Our words start to sound strange, nonlinear, emotional. Unpractical. Poetic. Once we have tasted this wildness, we begin to hunger for a food long denied us, and the more we eat the more we will awaken.[1]

Part of what we awaken to is the understanding that we are only individual in the sense that a mushroom is. The thing we call a mushroom, the fruiting body, is, indeed, a unique entity with a unique experience. But the "I" of the mushroom does not exist outside the "we" of the mycelium—which does not exist outside the "we" of the mycorrhizal network, which does not exist outside the "we" of the watershed. The same is true of each of us in relation to human and other-than-human community.

But to live in the light of that knowledge, we need to ground it in a web of relation we can directly experience. One way of doing that is by redefining our sense of sovereignty.

There has been a resurgence in recent years in remembering and recognizing that for ancient people sovereignty arose from the king wedding the spirit of the land. Unfortunately, much of what is being written and said about that wedding treats it as a private and metaphorical act performed by an individual to gain personal power and liberation. This reflects a profound misunderstanding.

In Irish culture, the rite by which the *rí* (king) wedded the land was not a solitary act, nor was it purely symbolic. The rite occurred in the presence of the entire *tuath* (tribe), and in many communities it was held at Samhain, the festival that marked the beginning of the dark half of the year, with the understanding that the dead, too, were witnessing and consecrating the marriage. The rí took on responsibilities on behalf of the community—not to rule in a modern sense but to unite the will of the people and, embodying that will, enter into a union with the sovereignty goddess as real as any human marriage. That sovereignty goddess was not an abstraction or an archetype; she was the living spirit of the land itself. And she alone had the right to bestow or revoke sovereignty from her bridegroom.

Certainly, in seeking to revive the spirit of this tradition in the modern world, there are aspects we can alter: the role of the rí need not be gendered in the way it was under ancient law, and how we define our tuath certainly must change in these times. My own approach to the latter question derives from John Moriarty's insight that a rí is "the dream of a people,"[2] and the people whom I ask to dream me are those human and other-than-human, living and dead, who join me in honoring the life of the land.

Ultimately, a rí requires a tuath and the tuath requires a rí. And the wedding vows require dedication in every moment and in every way to the land and the people. Sacral sovereignty is different from secular modern ideas of sovereignty as autonomy and self-direction. The rite fundamentally contradicts that cultural concept of uplifting the individual and making him accountable only to the self. Sacral sovereignty is a rite of devotion to communities, both human and wild. Only the living spirit of the land can choose who will wed her. But we can all cultivate the sense of love and devotion that marked the way of the rí. And in the absence of a tuath, we can call a community into being through building a practice that weaves relationships with our kin—living and dead, human and wild. Here are a few elements of such a practice.

CONNECT WITH YOUR ANCESTORS

Every animist culture that I am aware of honors its ancestors. And all of us are descended from animist cultures. Our neglected ancestors want to help us remember what they knew of the world.

Much has been written in recent years about ancestral trauma: about how traumatic experiences can change our DNA and how the impacts of trauma are thus passed down from one generation to the next. But if this is true (and it most definitely is), and if pleasure and joy and love shift our biochemistry as profoundly as sorrow and pain do (and they absolutely do), then aren't blessings and resilience also a part of our inheritance?

If you don't have the benefit of growing up in a living animist culture, one way to reorient to the world is to reach to the last ancestors who you are aware of who had an intact relationship with the living world around them. If you know your genealogy, look into the history and culture of the place where the oldest ancestors you are aware of lived, and trace that history back far enough to find what remnants exist of the customs and language and stories of people who experienced the world as alive and lived lives guided by the rhythms of the sun, the moon, the stars, and Earth. DNA tests can provide useful and intriguing information that might correct misremembered family origin stories or fill in gaps in information, but there are, of course, huge privacy concerns with them. If you don't know who your ancestors were, spend some time looking at photographs of different regions of the world and notice where you feel a resonance.

Make a small altar honoring your ancestors somewhere in your home. It can be simple to begin with: a picture or an object connected with the part of the world where they lived, a glass or cup to fill with water, and a small plate on which to make food offerings. Research the foods of that part of the world. Once a week, prepare one of those foods and sit down at the altar, giving a portion to the ancestors and a portion to yourself. If you eat with your family, it might be good to have an ancestor altar or altars in the room where you eat. Let your senses take in the scents and flavors and textures of the food and hold the intention of letting them awaken in you the things your ancestors would like you to remember.

Next, begin to look to language as a way of connecting with your ancestors. Sound resonates throughout our fascia and in our bones, and our bodies remember it deeply. From an early age, every time I have heard Irish Gaeilge spoken or sung—which, I think, may even have happened when my grandparents took me to meet my great uncle Jiggs, who played the squeezebox and was the first musician and first Irish speaker I ever met—I have felt myself shift into a different way of seeing the world, even without understanding a single word being spoken. The way words vibrate our vocal chords and echo in our chests when we speak or sing them also awakens ancestral memories in our bodies. I still have only enough Irish Gaeilge to make strange prayers and express stranger endearments, but speaking those words and phrases I have brings the feeling of my ancestors standing with me.

I recommend beginning with learning to say thank you in that language. As the great Christian mystic Meister Eckhart may have once said, "If the only prayer you said was 'thank you,' that would be enough." I know the divine by different names than he did, but gratitude is also the place where all my prayers begin. When I give thanks for my own life and the lives of my human and wild kin, I come into knowing my place in the world, and from there I can find the courses of action that will bring the greatest blessing to the community of life.

Learn what the words literally mean, and pay careful attention to everything you feel when you speak those words. *Go raibh míle maith agat* is the Irish way of saying "Thank you very much," but it literally means "May a thousand good things come toward you." Knowing that, when I speak the words, I feel the winds and currents that will carry all those good things to the person whose happiness I am praying for as I express my gratitude. Sometimes that "person" is an Oak or a Stag or a stone.

Once you have mastered a few simple phrases, see if you can learn a poem or a song that is meaningful to you in that language. A few years before he became poet laureate of the United States, I heard Robert Pinsky speak about how reading a poem aloud is an intimate act that connects you with everyone else who has ever read that poem aloud because you are all shaping the column of breath within your bodies in the same way. If you can, find the oldest stories available that are associated with your ancestors and tell them to people you love on dark winter nights. Then pay careful attention to your dreams.

Even if you do not know who your ancestors are, you can feel their echoes in your heartbeat and, through it, feed them gratitude. And the old, old, old ancestors whose hearts beat fluidly in response to the beating of the heart of the living world around them can teach us to shape the beats around the space in ways that allow the wild innocence at the center of the heart to sound through in the silence. To tap into this knowing, approach them in a way similar to the way I told you to approach a tree in chapter 1:

Take a deep breath and bring your attention a little to the left of your chest and feel for the beating of your heart.

Let its rhythm be your focus.

Before you were born, in the moments when it was first formed, across an ocean of amniotic fluid, your heart felt your mother's heart beating, and it stirred in response.

Just as her mother's heart stirred in response to her mother's heart.

And her mother's heart stirred in response to her mother's heart.

And her mother's heart stirred in response to her mother's heart. All the way back through the generations.

And no matter how painful, how confusing, how complex your relationship is to your mother or grandmother or great-grandmother, somewhere in that line of hearts is a heart that beats in perfect love and perfect trust, calling yours into resonance.

A heart untouched by trauma. A heart untouched by guilt and shame and fear.

Feel for it. Feel back through the lineage of heartbeats. Through the generations. And let your heart meet and match its rhythm.

Let that rhythm guide you to coherence.

From that place of coherence, begin the work of remaking the world.

HONOR THE SUN

Victor Anderson said that the sun is the god of this solar system.[3] The sun is the source of nourishment for the plants that give us oxygen and thus also for the lives of animals and fungi who feed on the bodies of plants and on each other. It is the source of our metabolic fires and for the fires of the furnaces we build.

By shining through our skin and our skulls, it also shines onto our pituitary glands and our pineal glands, guiding their release of hormones that orchestrate the actions of the rest of our bodies' organs. Philosopher, bodyworker, and anatomist Gil Hedley says that the sun is our master endocrine gland.[4]

Honor the sun by bringing your attention and gratitude to it when you wake, at noon, and at sunset.

HONOR THE WATERS

Water is central to my cosmology and to the cosmology of my ancestors, as this book has made clear. Water is also what we are mostly made of and what plants are mostly made of.

Find out where the water you drink comes from. Once a week, if it is nearby—and once a season, if it is far from you—bring a simple offering to the water and say thank you in one of your ancestral languages. I personally favor whiskey, honey, and milk as offerings.

Find a place where there is wild water near you. Once a week spend at least half an hour gazing at the water and bringing your focus back to the sight and sound of the water every time your attention wanders. Find out what watershed you live in—the place where the water that falls on the ground flows to. Regularly bring offerings of purifying herbs to that water. Find out what threatens the health of the waters of your home and find what you can do to protect and restore them.

Begin each day with a glass of water and the words *thank you*.

HONOR THE TREES

Find the oldest trees that share the land with you. Once a week bring offerings to each and sit and listen to them.

Find the youngest trees that share the land with you. Once a week bring them water and tell them the things you want future generations, human and wild, to remember of the times we are living in.

PRACTICE WILD HOSPITALITY

In modern Irish, the word *flaithiúlacht* suggests kindness and generosity. In earlier times, when hospitality was one of the most important cultural values, it was synonymous with nobility.

How can you show flaithiúlacht to your wild kin? Take the time to learn what the water, the soil, the plants, the fungi need to survive and thrive. Do all that is in your power to help them meet their needs Find out who is missing from your ecological community and what would be needed for those beings to return. Do whatever is in your power to make that possible. And whether or not is not within your power to help them in a material way, bring the present and absent members of your ecological community to the awareness of your heart every day.

MARK THE SEASONS

As I said when writing about the Cauldron of Motion, my teacher, Cornelia Benavidez, recently reminded me that people around the world have always marked seasonal changes and the cycles of the sun, the moon, and the stars with shared work, feasting, and ritual. What do you do if you don't already mark these cycles in your life?

One thing you can do is look to your ancestral traditions of marking the seasons—but the seasons where you are might be different from the seasons where your ancestors lived. It is still well worth looking for elements of their seasonal rituals that might be incorporated into your own; this will deepen your connection with them.

The best thing to do is to make a point of walking in the same forest once a week, every week for a year. Keep track of the changes you feel in your body and the changes you witness in the forest and look up (or, better yet, observe) what is happening with the sun, the moon, the stars, and the weather. Notice the big turning points, when changes in your body and changes in the land quicken. These will be the points you will choose for next year's celebration. Note as many of the changes taking place in these times as you can, and look for the energetic nature of the shifts the pattern of signs indicates.

The following year, during each of those major turning points, invite friends to do some work with you outdoors that is fitting for the season and then share a meal of seasonal, local food. Do this every year.

Now, let me introduce my own seasonal ritual cycle that combines the calendar of my ancestors with my experiences of living in northern New England.

Our Lady of the Apples
drinks in the fermentation
of her own fallen fruit,
slipping into slumber
beneath the snow.

She will wake at Bealtaine,
clothed in white blossoms,
shimmering promise
of sweetness to come.

7

The Wheel of the Year

The ways in which we measure and experience time play in important role in how we relate to each other and to the living world. Our dominant culture views time in a linear, progressive way—a process that is always moving forward. When we ourselves approach time in that way, we push ourselves forward until we can push no more. We are horses with blinders on being driven down a path not of our making without regard to the landscape it moves through. And this changes our sense of what healing means—instead of seeking a wholeness that mirrors the balance of a healthy ecology, we seek to remove obstacles to our linear progress, often at our own peril.

Most every preindustrial culture viewed time in a cyclical way and aligned the rhythms of individual and community life with the rhythms of life itself revealed in the seasonal patterns of animals, plants, weather, water, and land and of the sun, moon, and stars above. Even medieval Christianity with its liturgical calendar of holy days celebrating saints whose lives and stories were tied to particular times and places maintained these deep, old rhythms. Modern Catholicism holds onto this to some degree, but outside a few rural places in Europe and Latin America, this is mostly only true in the lives of priests, monks, and nuns and is often devoid of the local specificity it had in the Middle Ages, which tied people to the land. It is no accident that the Protestant elimination of holy days and holy places coincided with the rise of capitalism.

Approaching time in a cyclical way, working with a Wheel of the Year, is an important part of much of modern Pagan practice, but many contemporary people miss the deeper purpose and meaning woven into the structure of this wheel. My friend and teacher Cornelia Benavidez recently told me about the Wheel of the Year.

Ask any modern Pagan about the Wheel of the Year, and you will hear pretty much the same thing: that it is all about seasonal change and fertility rites. Yes, this is a part of it, but it is also so much more. Both Victor Anderson and Margaret Korwin (two of my teachers in the Craft) told me that the ways of Indigenous people all around the world throughout our ancient ancestral histories found creative ways of developing complete and thoughtful ways of looking at the reality around them. They observed and sought out various ways of communing with nature by becoming an active part of its cycles. As humankind became more refined by wanting and gaining answers to all sorts of questions, they grew in complexity, and people turned within as well as reached out to the divine source that had birthed consciousness itself. Through observations and experiences, we bonded closer to each other creating celebrations and rituals. This brought us closer together as people and closer to all that is alive around us, seen and unseen. The wheel and all the holidays remind us and teach us about order, respect, and thankfulness for the land and for the skills of nature and to appreciate the reflection of that within ourselves so that we know that we are not alone but a part of something wondrous. This is the life that inspires us, drives us to be creative and, by doing so, to touch the divine inside ourselves and strive to learn and grow in an ever-evolving world. It is here that we find meaning, inner strength, and emotional discipline. It is here that innocence finds peace and protection to grow into wisdom. Here, we gain the clarity and skills to become artisans, healers, and teachers of a balanced path connected to the past and present. This is what can sustain a healthy culture for the future.

Those of us who did not receive an intact transmission of a healthy culture—especially those of us whose last animist ancestors lived in distant lands—find ourselves with the task of trying to create one. With luck and blessing, we will have the opportunity to pass it down to those with whom we share common values—whether they be children who are part of our lives or people of younger generations outside our families with whom we share a deep kinship. Central to the creation or revitalization of a culture is the evolution of the calendar that shapes the rhythms of its people's lives.

What follows is a description of the cyclical rhythms that guide my own life. I mark time primarily by the four fire festivals of my Irish ancestors: Samhain, Imbolc, Bealtaine, and Lughnassadh. I mark these festivals in ways that combine elements of Irish tradition, elements of the traditions Cornelia Benavidez taught me, and personal elements that arise from my own relationship to the mountains and forest I call home.

It begins, as all things do, in darkness.

SAMHAIN

The nights grow long and cold, as leaf and fruit fall to
the ground, plants reach into the darkness as they once
reached for the light, sending life down into their roots.
All winter, they will dream beneath the earth.

As the life above the ground retreats beneath it, the fungal life beneath the ground, the mycelial webs that intertwine with rhizomes to form the mind of the forest, send up new life, the fruiting bodies of mushrooms. In the shadow of Birches and Pines, *Amanita* mushrooms burst forth, bearing the bright yellow of another season's sunlight, the red that is the color of the lifeblood, speckled with the white of the Otherworld. To the peoples of Northern Europe, who knew how to avoid being poisoned, these mushrooms were a sacrament, a bringer of bright vision in a dark season.

The mushrooms both bring and are brought by the autumn rains. Summer lightning proliferated the tendrils of the mycelium, bringing life to the land. October rains bring their fruiting. The structure of the mushrooms creates microclimates beneath and around them, conjuring their own winds to carry the spores they release up into the atmosphere where water condenses around them, becoming clouds. The trees whose rhizomes intertwine with the mycelium that gives rise to the mushrooms reach upward for water and pull it down. The rains water the soil dried by the long, hot summer and nourish root, seed, and mycelium alike. Soon the snow will blanket them, keeping them warm and protected through the long winter and watering them anew in the spring.

Across the ocean from my home in western Maine, in the Oak and Yew forests on the shores of Lough Lein, in the weeks before now the Red Deer Stags adorned their antlers with branches, Ferns, and moss, making crowns for their season of battle and of courtship. Now the Fawns gestate in the wombs of the Does. And on both sides of the ocean, now is the season of the hunt, of the culling of the herd, the blood harvest that ensures that the forest on which the herd depends will not be stripped away to nothing before spring. Each life-form, be it plant, animal, fungal, or bacterial, depends directly or indirectly on the death of other life and in time repays the debt incurred by returning to the earth, the dead life-form's molecules in time finding form as new life.

The Bear goes into the womb of Earth to prepare for winter dreaming. In this same season the filidh, the prophet-poets of my ancestors, would go into wild places and dark caves and scry on smooth waters to seek the kind of vision that can come only in the dark of the year.

The Old Irish year began and ended in this dark time—just as all things begin and end in darkness: our own lives, the life of our sun, the life of all the worlds. Many modern Pagans mark the old festival of Samhain on October 31, the date appropriated by the Catholic Church to be All Hallows' Eve. That appropriation came before the imposition of the Gregorian calendar, so the old rites were likely once observed closer to November 11 and still are by custom in some parts of Ireland. By a still older reckoning, the festival came at the time when the Pleiades were at their apex in the night sky.

In this world, Samhain marked the beginning of the dark half of the year and the end of its bright half. The last fruit was on the Blackthorn, the Hawthorn, and the Rowan. What root crops remained in the ground and what grains remained in the field were a tithe to the Otherworld. So were the bones of Deer and Cattle thrown on the great fires atop the high hills. I honor the custom from Connemara in the west of Ireland of harvesting nothing from forest or field from Samhain until the end of winter—though I make exception for fallen branches, fallen lichens, and resins flowing freely from trees.

In the Otherworld, the Hawthorn blooms with its scent of sex and death, the white blossoms of the Blackthorn come where leaves will follow, and a silver Apple tree bears both flowers and golden fruit at once. In the Otherworld, it is Bealtaine, the time of life's stirring and springing forth. The Hawthorn's scent conveys the truth that Bealtaine and Samhain are two sides of the same coin, the currency of life's shape-shifting continuation.

This world and the Otherworld are not always apart. Recounting a fundamental aspect of a dying worldview that infused life in rural Ireland, Manchán Magan, a journalist dedicated to preserving and revitalizing vanishing parts of the Irish language, writes:

Ceantar means place, region, or locality, while *alltar* is its opposite: the other realm, the netherworld. In the Irish mindset the *ceantar* is closely shadowed by the *alltar*. They exist simultaneously in all places, at all times. Our physical bodies occupy the *ceantar*, but our minds can easily slip into the *alltar*.

This idea that there were different levels beneath and between what we could see was once so widely accepted that it didn't even deserve mentioning, but nowadays the word *alltar* has almost disappeared. Only a thin veil separated the two realms, *ceantar* and *alltar* and there were always those who could pass from one to the other.[1]

That veil was the spell of Manannán, god of the sea, cast to separate the worlds when the Tuath Dé, the Tribe of the Gods, left this world when newcomers to the land brought ways too brutal and regimented for them. Some are able to see or move through this cloak of mist at will; some are taken across it by the Daoine Sidhe, the people the Tuath Dé became when they went into the ancient burial mounds all across the Irish countryside, which also served as ritual chambers, always facing westward toward the open ocean and into a realm in which time moves differently. But it is most easily breached in both directions at Samhain (and at Bealtaine). Robin Artisson writes:

> On Samhain, all of the worlds, and therefore, all beings, are mystically returned to the time of old night, the state the Greeks might have called "chaos," the mystery that existed before the birth of the universe. . . . The power of the Samhain season destroys the metaphysical barriers between the living and the dead, and so for one sacred period, there at the time of the death and renewal of the year and the cosmos, the entire "clan" or kin-group can truly be together, living and dead.[2]

The living members of the tribe, their ancestors, and their descendants, yet to be born, were united by the figure of the rí, the sacral king. The rí was not a monarch in the modern sense—not a maker of laws, or even of decisions—the law was encoded in *seanchas* (the body of lore containing history, genealogy, and customs) and interpreted by legal specialists called *brehons*. Decisions were made by tribal assemblies over which the rí presided. The role of the rí was a priestly or shamanic role: he was the one who embodied the community's connection to the land, and the one who would rally the people on the battlefield when the land and the tribe needed to be protected. This bond was solidified at Samhain, when the rí was ritually wedded to the land. This is also the mating season of the Red Deer, whose Stag has long been a symbol of the sacral king in both Gaelic and

Brythonic cultures. The Fawns conceived in this season will be born in the season of Bealtaine.

The spirit of the land was said to come to the rí first as the Cailleach—a word that means "hag" or "crone" in modern Irish, but originally meant "veiled woman." The veil that she wore was the face of terror. If the man who would be rí rejected her or fled, the land itself would reject him, and death or exile would be his fate. But if he kissed her, the veil lifted, and she became a shimmering vision of beauty, her scent and the taste of her lips bringing sweet intoxication.

That wedding at Samhain marked a gift of fertility from this world to the Otherworld—a gift that would be returned in May, when life flows from the Otherworld below up into this world.

To be wedded to the land is to understand that life and death, beauty and terror, bride and bridegroom are inextricably linked. None can exist without the other. To know the light that is to come, we must first love the darkness from which it will emerge, just as seed and root find comfort in the soil where they wait for the sun to stir them to life in spring.

✦ Samhain Ritual ✦

Fill a bowl with water. Ideally, water from a spring or well, but any clean water will do.

Go outside beneath the stars. Light a candle and a smudge or incense. Angelica, or another aromatic root, is ideal.

If you can recognize the Pleiades, look up at them. If you cannot, just ask in your heart that they shine into the water.

Hold the intention that the ancestors who knew how to live with Earth in harmony will give you guidance.

Bring your attention to your heartbeat, and then to your root, and then to the subtle cord that runs from your heart through your root and to the center of Earth. With a soft-focus gaze into the bowl, notice the feelings and sensations and thoughts that arise.

When you are done, thank the stars and the ancestors, and pour the water out onto the land.

IMBOLC

The darkness is deep in winter in Maine, and so is the snow. During the brief hours of daylight, the scents of Pine, Fir, and Spruce fill the crisp, cold air. Beneath the snow, most plants slumber, the embers of life held in roots that hold the nourishment made by the light·of a season gone by.

With Imbolc, at the beginning of February, the lengthening of the days, which have been growing longer since the Winter Solstice, becomes more pronounced. The winter sun begins to stir something in us. But the night is still dark. In Ireland, the first wildflowers come at this time of year. Here in Maine, we will have no visible signs of spring until March when warm days and cold nights set first the Maple and then the Birch sap to running and Skunk Cabbage melts through the ice, soon to draw hungry bears from their dreaming.

The most likely etymology of Imbolc is the Old Irish word *imbolc*, which means "in the belly." In this season, the Fawn grows in the womb of the Doe, and seeds held in the belly of Earth feel the hint of the sun's warmth.

Sometime after the coming of Christianity to Ireland, Imbolc became syncretized with Saint Brighid's Day. We have only fragments of knowledge about who Brighid of the Tuath Dé was to pre-Christian Irish people, nor do we know whether they honored her at this time of year. But whether or not Imbolc was her festival prior to the sixth century, her presence this time of year becomes palpable to me, and her qualities are reflected in those of the saint the Irish church honors on the first of February.

The idea of a saint and a goddess being incarnations of the same spirit would not have been strange to my Irish ancestors in the first centuries after Christianity. Gods were ancestors who had mastered a powerful magic during their lives and sometimes were born again in different generations. Saints were ancestors who had performed miracles and learned to embody holy mysteries. Sometimes the merging of saint and a god into one person was made explicit. Lí Ban, sister of Fand, who came to this world from the Plain of Honey as a Bird, was drowned beneath a lake and became half Salmon and swam to the sea where she was caught in a fishing net by a monk who brought her to his abbot Comgall who baptized her as Muirgead, "Sea Born." She is now a saint whose feast day is January 27.

The goddess Brighid is a daughter of the Dagda and a great poet. She, or two sisters of hers who bore the same name, was or were also a great physician and a gifted smith. She was and is connected both to sacred wells (as we discussed earlier in this book) and with fire. I know her as the keeper of three bright flames—the fire of inspiration, the fire of healing, and the fire of transformation.

The red-eared Cow, the Ewe, the Cockerel, the herald of the new day, and, in Scotland, the Snake, symbol of healing and regeneration, the creature whose body always kisses the earth, are all associated with Brighid. She has an even older association with the Swan—a bird of beauty, grace, and power. The first priests and shamans of Europe wore Swan feather cloaks, which gave way to the feathered cloaks of the filidh, the prophet-poets who Brighid guided and protected.

Saint Brighid was the daughter of a Pagan chieftain who became a midwife for Mary and then returned to Ireland to found a monastery in Kildare (Cill Dara or Church of the Oak, a tree connected with the Dagda). She is a patron saint of poets, midwives, healers, blacksmiths, cattle, and holy wells. Nuns devoted to her have kept a sacred flame burning in Kildare for centuries, and some say they were preceded by priestesses who kept a flame for her Pagan namesake.

Samhain is focused on connection with the Otherworld; Imbolc is focused on surviving the winter in this world. Brighid's rites at this time of year are connected with blessing the hearth and the home.

On the eve of Saint Brighid's Day, in many parts of Ireland, people traditionally put a cloth outside at sunset, the Brat Bride, Brighid's Cloak, which they bring inside in the morning and use in prayers for healing throughout the rest of the coming year. In many areas, a bed of

Birch twigs and Rushes was traditionally prepared for a doll, the *brideog*, who represented Brighid. Children would later take the doll from house to house, bringing Brighid's blessing and receiving gifts of milk, cheese, and butter. An evening feast rich with these foods would traditionally be followed by the whole family spending the evening by the fire weaving solar crosses from Rushes to bless the home and all who dwell within it with health and prosperity for the coming year. Robin Artisson writes:

> Brigid, the sweet Goddess of inspiration and all of the arts and crafts is especially venerated at this time, because in the grip of darkness and cold, we need our spirits and hopes renewed. She is also there to prepare us with the skills and inspiration we need to face the year and get the many tasks of the year done. When Brigid manifests in her many fires in this season, we see the Old Veiled One become young again, in a way—we see the breaking of darkness with pure light and the dangerous forces of the land and the Sidhe will no longer be a threat to us.[3]

He notes that this is also a time of purification by fire and water—beginning to move what has attached to us or stagnated within us all winter in preparation for spring. Purification in the sense of clearing away whatever blocks the flow of vitality. We clear the way to come back into our bodies and into the living world, carrying the insights of winter's long dreaming, just as the sap begins to flow in the Maple and the Birch, bringing the gift of sweetness in the weeks to come.

🌿 Imbolc Ritual 🌿

The night before your ritual, leave a white altar cloth outside. Bring it in when you wake.

Put out an offering for Brighid. Honey, milk, and whiskey are traditional and combine quite nicely.

Set out three candles, and place a bowl of water in front of each.

As you light the first candle, ask for the fire of the hearth to warm your cauldron of incubation. Gaze into the water and ask what is needed to nourish your life and the life of the land.

As you light the second candle, ask the fire of the forge to heat your cauldron of motion. Gaze into the water and ask how you can best shape the rhythms of your life to be in harmony with the life of the land.

As you light the third candle, ask the fire of inspiration to warm the cauldron of wisdom and spark the fire in your head. Gaze into the water and ask how you can inspire people to live in ways that honor the land.

Let the candles burn down.

Pour the offerings out onto the land.

BEALTAINE

The ice is slowly melting from the lake. Snow is still thick on the ground, but Blackbirds fill the branches of the budding Alders.

The Blackbirds among the Alders at the water's edge were a sign of life returning to the land for my Irish ancestors as well. A poem attributed to Fionn MacCumhaill, the boy who caught the Salmon of Knowledge and grew to become a great warrior, written sometime between the ninth and eleventh centuries, begins:

> *May-day, season surpassing!*
> *Splendid is colour then.*
> *Blackbirds sing a full lay,*
> *If there be a slender shaft of day.*[4]

My first time in Ireland, lying on wet earth, amid a grove of Alder trees, I had a vision. First I saw the shape of an Alder leaf and saw it become the shield of a warrior king. Then I saw myself as that king, returning from battle, and being brought to a warrior woman who was the protector of a holy well. She sent everyone else away and tended to me herself. As she leaned in, I looked deeply into her green eyes and heard the words "Only she who has swum in dark waters can hold he who has gazed into the Abyss."

I knew almost nothing about Alder then, but the more I learn about Alder, the more that vision makes sense. I lived for three years in a place where Alders lined the water's edge. Every day, I passed through them when I brought my kayak to the water, where I paddled out into the middle of the cove, focused on the reflection of the Alders, Birches, Spruce, and Fir in the still water, and soon felt the presence of She Who Dwells Below, an older, wilder version of the one some call the Lady of the Lake. She looked at me with those same green eyes. They are the same green as the leaves that grow on the Alder in the season to come.

The Irish name for May Day is Lá Bealtaine. It sits opposite Samhain on the Wheel of the Year. The Otherworld is close at hand, bringing an infusion of life, a bursting forth of green into our world. At Samhain, the Hawthorn and the Blackthorn bloomed in the Otherworld. Now they bloom in hedgerows and around sacred wells and atop the hills and mounds that they guard. Before the Catholic Church brought the Roman calendar, Bealtaine began when the Hawthorn bloomed. In the seanchas, the old lore, it is a day associated with the beginning of one world and the ending of another. The Hawthorn bloomed on the day that the Tuath Dé arrived in ships that sailed the sky, riding the black north wind. The Hawthorn bloomed again on the day that the Tuath Dé lost their world, when Amergin stood atop the sacred hill of Uisneach and chanted the song that created a new, human, civilized world atop the old world of the Shining Ones.

In Ireland, wildflowers bloom. Here in Maine, life stirs beneath the snow, and in the coming weeks the Trout Lily and the Trillium will emerge. In forests on both sides of the Atlantic, the Deer who mated in autumn give birth.

Bealtaine is a time of fertility. The blessing the sacral king poured into the land when he made love with the goddess of sovereignty at Samhain becomes the green of emerging life. Green is the color of the mantle worn by those who pass between worlds. And as the red of our blood, from the oxidized iron in our hemoglobin, is the color of human life, the green of chlorophyll, a molecule similar to hemoglobin that contains magnesium instead of iron, is the color of life in the plant kingdom.

For my Irish ancestors, the focus of Bealtaine rituals was on the fertility of the land and the protection of livestock. It was a time of blessing and purification by fire, mirroring the growing power of the sun and initiating the beginning of the bright half of the year.

For many modern Pagans, the focus of Bealtaine is on celebrating the holiness, beauty, and joy of human sexuality and its relationship to the blossoming of Earth. Some reconstructionists and historians criticize this focus as ahistorical. But need our celebrations be historical? We live in a different cultural and historical context than our ancestors did.

Until Norman invaders, backed by papal authority, imposed Catholicism as we know it on Ireland—a religion later outlawed by the Norman's British descendants in favor of compulsory Protestantism during their occupation of the country—sexual shame was not a part of Christianity in Ireland, nor was it an element of pre-Christian Irish culture. Early Irish Christianity also incorporated Pagan reverence for the living world. Human sexuality and the fertility of the land were not separated from each other in people's worldviews or in their lived experience, so there was no need to reinforce or reiterate their connection.

This is decidedly not the case in the dominant culture in North America today. On the one hand, a Puritanical strain to the culture fills many with deep shame about their sexuality. On the other hand, the commodification first of bodies and then of images of bodies creates a strange kind of erotic dissociation so that for many people sexuality becomes an imitation of pornographic simulations of someone else's fantasies. Puritanism and pornography both de-eroticize and desecrate sexuality and human bodies, so we have a need to resanctify the erotic and reconnect it with the fertility of Earth.

What does this mean? In an interview with Derek Jensen, ecofeminist writer Terry Tempest Williams said:

Erotic means "in relation." Erotic is what those deep relations are and can be that engage the whole body—our heart, our mind, our spirit, our flesh. It is that moment of being exquisitely present. It does not speak well for us as a people that we even have to make the distinction between what is erotic and what is not, because an erotic connection is a life-engaged making love to the world that I think comes very naturally.[5]

In a healthy culture, eros pervades our relationship with the living world—not just our intimate relationships with other people. The feeling is stirred by the grace of a lithe Birch, by the magnificence of an ancient Oak, by the power of waves crashing against a rocky cliff, by the sublime beauty of mountains and forests reflected in still water, by the way a horse moves is felt in the body—in the ways it changes heartbeat and breath, stirs the movement of blood, and awakens every nerve ending. It is a feeling not only of awe but also of connection, connection that brings meaning. It is erotic in the oldest, truest sense of the word. You can be celibate or asexual and still experience this kind of eros, but you cannot curse or debase your own sexuality or your own body without also impacting your ability to feel this erotic connection with all of life.

The virility and fecundity of the land is the source of our own virility and fecundity. Bealtaine is in invitation to open our hearts and our roots to the green and blossoming life of the world, that we too might flower in the fullness of who we are, rooted in Earth.

⚘ Bealtaine Ritual ⚘

Fill a bowl with water. Ideally, water from a spring or well, but any clean water will do.

Go outside at dawn or at noon and hold the water up toward the sun.

Hold the intention that the life awakening in the land move through you.

Bring your attention to your heartbeat, and then to your root, and then to the subtle cord that runs from your heart through your root and to the center of Earth. As you inhale, draw the green force of life up through your root into your heart. With a soft-focus gaze into the bowl, notice the feelings and sensations and thoughts that arise.

Gently put the bowl down onto the ground, and let your body find the movement that arises from the feelings stirred within you.

When you are done, give thanks. Pour half the water onto the earth and drink the other half.

LUGHNASSADH

The sun blazed brightly at noon, but as the day pro-
gresses, the Tansy and Yarrow dance in the cold wind
that blows from the West, bringing in rain. In the fields,
St. John's Wort is fading, giving way to Goldenrod. In the
early mornings, Bears gorge on Blueberries in the fields
up the road, while in the forest the Blueberry's strange
Otherworldly cousin, Ghost Pipe, blooms, and across
the ocean in my ancestral homeland, the hillsides are
purple with Heather. The Rowan is laden with berries.

Lughnassadh, or Lúnasa in modern Irish, means "assembly of Lugh," the ancient fire festival that marks the harvest of the first fruits and grains and the beginning of summer's dying into winter. Between now and Samhain, flowers will give way to fruit and seeds, the leaves of all but the evergreens will die and fall away, and plants will sink their energy and their consciousness down into their roots. This is a time for celebrating and giving thanks for the harvest—but also for taking stock of what is at hand and what must be preserved and put away. What must be let go, and what must be planted in autumn to bring forth new life in spring.

The seanchas, the old lore, the stories and genealogies and histories and laws that made the Irish a people, tells us that the festival that marks the day was begun by Lugh—sun-bright, long-armed, many-skilled king of the Tuath Dé—to honor his foster mother, Tailitu, of the axe, the plain, the great labor, who died of exhaustion after clearing forests to make way for fields of grain. Lugh was a great warrior and magician who played a key role in helping the Tuath Dé liberate Ireland from Balor of the Baleful Eye, whose gaze corrupted everything it landed on. (John Moriarty notes that the gaze of our contemporary culture, which commodifies everything it sees, is the modern equivalent of Balor's Baleful Eye.)

Tailitu herself was a woman of the Fir Bolg, the People of the Thunder God, a people who lived alongside the Tuath Dé. Both suffered under the oppression of Balor's people, the Fomorians, who demanded sacrifice and tribute. It was the ancestral forest of her own people that Tailitu cleared that it might bring forth plentiful harvests of grain—grain that would be taxed by their oppressors.

This story gives way to another old name for this time of year, *Brón Trogain*. *Brón* means "sorrow," and *trogain* is an Old Irish word with three primary meanings. In applying each to the name of the season, we can gain another layer of understanding. In one meaning, Brón Trogain translates to "sorrow of the land." Why does the land grieve? She grieves for the life-forms that must die each season; fruit and grain must fall to the ground to become the source of new life in spring. This season, she tells me she grieves for the destruction of the forests that came before the fields. She grieves that her children, the plants and animals, live in bondage under the rule of people who do not respect them or her.

Brón Trogain also has an association with the Raven. The modern Irish name for Raven is *fiach dubh*, meaning "black debt," which I connect with the grim price paid when battle, physical or metaphysical, becomes the cost of defending sovereignty. A scavenger on the battlefield, Raven reminds us that we owe our life and our very flesh to the living world around us. A nineteenth-century German dictionary of Old Irish connects the word *trogan*, of which *trogain* is the genitive form, with the Gothic German word *tabenweibchen*, meaning "wife of the Raven." While Irish tradition has no references to the Raven's wife, there is a prominent and powerful Irish goddess connected with the Raven. The Raven is the bird of the Morrigan, who many today think of as the Irish goddess of war, but I think of more as the dark face of the sovereignty goddess, who reflects the grim price her people pay for their freedom. While there is no traditional lore that I am aware of connecting her with this time of year, when I reflect on this meaning of Brón Trogain, I feel her grief for the blood that has watered her fields instead of rain, for the loss of life, for the indignity of bondage, for the deaths of the sacral kings who had given their lives for her and for her people, and for the lack of true sovereigns in the generations since they perished.

It brings to mind Seamus Heaney's devastatingly beautiful poem "Requiem for the Croppies,"[6] which mourns the Irish who died fighting for independence in the uprising of 1798. They knew that English forces would not afford them a proper burial, so they filled their coat pockets with Barley so that the places they fell would not be unmarked. The last of the rebels were slaughtered at Vinegar Hill in Wexford that June. Speaking as the voice of those fallen ones, Heaney writes:

> *Terraced thousands died, shaking scythes at cannon.*
> *The hillside blushed, soaked in our broken wave.*
> *They buried us without shroud or coffin*
> *And in August . . . the barley grew up out of our grave.*

The green and gold of the Barley that year were the colors of a harvest of sorrow that nevertheless brought forth new life. And it is from Barley that *uisce beatha*, "the water of life," known in English as whiskey, is distilled over a peat fire whose smoke carries the ancient exhalations of the forests and meadows that became the bogs where the peat was formed and where sometimes offerings to the gods were left and preserved—butter, wooden carvings, bodies of the dead. The juice of the Barley brings warmth in winter.

Finally, Brón Trogain means "labor pains." It may seem paradoxical to speak of birth in a season when things are dying back, but late summer is the season when plants are focused on bringing forth fruit and seed. Most modern Pagans think of Bealtaine as the season of fertility, but more properly speaking, we experience attraction and pleasure and flowering and pollination in spring, while it is autumn that the forest and field are fecund. Fecundity and fertility are the maturation of the friskiness of spring. Lughnassadh is the time of fruition.

🍃 Lughnassadh Ritual 🍃

Lay a red or gold cloth on your altar. Fill two plates with fruits and edible seeds from the season's harvest and place them to the left and right sides of the altar.

In the middle of your altar, place three bowls of water from a spring, a well, or a wild stream. Place a candle, preferably a beeswax candle, by each bowl, on the side of the bowl farthest from you.

Light the first candle, and ask: What died that we might live, that we might have this harvest, and how shall we honor it? Gaze into the water until you feel you have learned the answer.

Light the second candle, and ask: What labor of ours will this harvest nourish that will help give life to the world to come? Gaze into the water until you feel you have learned the answer.

Light the third candle, and ask: What seeds shall we plant in the burned-over soils that forest and meadow might grow again? Gaze into the water until you feel you have learned the answer.

When you are done with this divination work, call up a feeling of gratitude for the harvest, and eat from the plate on the right side of your altar. When you are done, extinguish the candles. Pour the water from each bowl out onto the earth. Take the plate from the left of your altar and leave it in a place where birds and other wild animals might find it until sunset of the following day.

The Corn surrenders to the Crow
giving its ghost to become
the wings and feathers
that will carry the seed
to new soil,

The Apple lets go the burden of its fruit,
which ferments in the fading sunlight,
that the roots might drink it in
as the season of slumber approaches,

Fallen leaves feed the mycelium
brought to life by the lightning
the Oak called down in summer,

The King accepts the Cailleach's kiss
and approaches the threshold
of the stone chamber
where all winter he will shift shape
from Salmon to Bear to forest to man
and emerge again in spring
to bring life to the Dream of the Land.

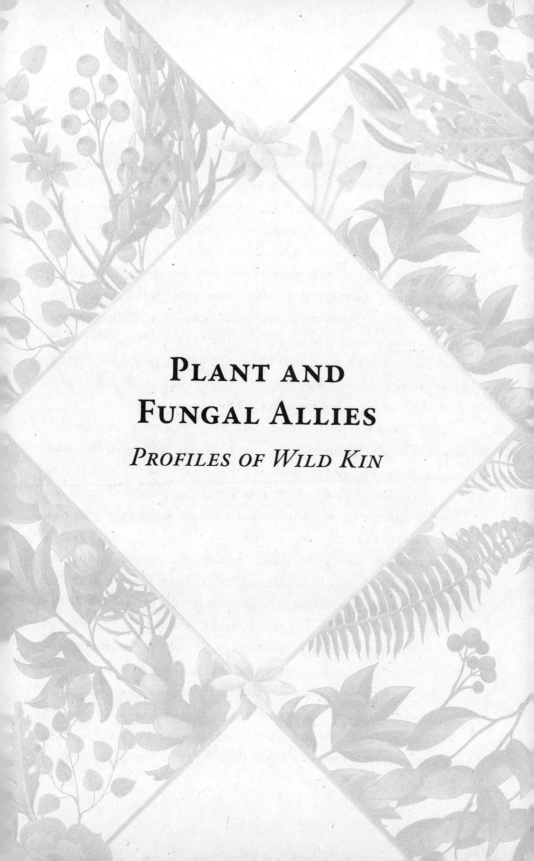

PLANT AND
FUNGAL ALLIES

PROFILES OF WILD KIN

What does it mean to call a plant an ally? As a poet and a witch, I believe that words used with precision have great power to shape someone's experience of the world. The word *ally* comes from the Old French *alier,* meaning "to join in marriage." Originally a verb, the word was first used as a noun in the fourteenth century to mean "kin." It speaks of intimacy, tenderness, and trust. A deep knowing.

It begins with coming to know a plant on its own terms. Getting down on the ground and sitting with the plant. Coming back to it again and again. Coming to know the way the light shines on the plant at different times of day. The scent of the soil where it grows. The way the air tastes around the plant. Coming to know the body of the plant the way you would come to know the body of a lover. Knowing the feeling of its leaves and petals against your skin. Coming to love the ways it curves toward the sun.

And it requires getting quiet enough to notice what the plant stirs in you. The subtle sensations in your body. The memories, emotions, images, scents, and snatches of music that come to you. The ways your dreams change. Like a lover or a dear friend, a plant will teach you things you didn't know about yourself, new ways of being in your own body, new ways of being in the world.

Don't make the mistake of thinking that what you are learning and experiencing is all in your head. Don't think that to speak of a plant in the same terms you would use to describe a beloved is to lie and think and speak in metaphor. If you treat any of this as a metaphor, you will miss out on the chance to experience this other being in all of its magnificence—and to see your own beauty and power from the perspective of the plant.

But when coming to know a plant truly mirrors, in every way, the process of falling in love, everything changes. The idea of the world as sacred and alive opens into the experience of a world in which another consciousness embodied in a wildly different form from your own can speak directly to your heart.

Being Present with Plants

To listen to a plant with your heart, go back to the technique in chapter 1, which I learned from Stephen Buhner and Julie McIntyre, for a connecting with a tree. I summarize it again here.

Bring your attention to the beating of your own heart. As you feel your heartbeat, think of how your heart has beat for you in every moment of your life, through wild joy and deep sorrow, without your ever needing to ask it to. Let gratitude arise like a wild spring from the center of your heart and fill it. Bless your blood, so that it flows throughout your body and comes out with your breath, blessing the world. Let that gratitude come back in with your next in-breath.

With your next inhalation, feel that gratitude coming in with your breath, flowing toward your heart. Let your attention expand from your heart down to your root. Let your awareness move from your own root down into the soil and grow tendrils that intertwine with the roots and rhizomes of the plant you seek to connect with.

Now allow yourself to feel the presence of the plant. Allow images, sensations, scents, memories, fragments of song, to arise. Be present with them without yet attempting to assign them meaning.

When you are ready, thank the plant, and then draw your awareness back up through your root to your heart. Pay attention again to your own heartbeat and thank your heart. Run your hands over your own body, with a firm touch, letting yourself feel your boundaries and your solidity. Take some time to record and reflect on what you experienced and learned.

Having connected intimately in this way, the utilitarian view of the plant falls away. The answer to the question "What is Skunk Cabbage good for?" shifts from "Skunk Cabbage is good for calming spasms and clearing fluid from the lungs" to "Skunk Cabbage is good for setting roots deep in the mud and melting its way through the ice to blossom forth in a gorgeous purple flower." Or "Skunk Cabbage is good for being Skunk Cabbage."

And the quality of the medicine and magic you work with the plant changes as well—the plant goes from being an inert substance chosen according to memorized sets of indications and properties and correspondences to being an active participant in shared work. New ways of working with the plant will emerge from your relationship.

And the relationship will demand of you consistency and honor, something else Stephen Buhner taught me about. You will find yourself compelled to keep commitments you have made to spend time with the plant. And your respect for the plant will grow from an intellectual belief in the importance of avoiding overharvesting to a deep personal investment in seeing the plant flourish and defending the places it calls home.

This is not a path for the faint of heart. Like any intimate relationship, a true alliance with a plant will make you look at aspects of your life—patterns of thought and feeling and action—that you would rather ignore. And unbound by human etiquette, plants, like gods, will not change the subject or gloss things over with niceties and half-truths.

To deeply meet and be deeply met by a consciousness that exists so far outside the ideas and beliefs and stories and ideologies and hangups of our culture is to be seduced into wandering out through a gap in the crumbling wall around our civilization and into the borderlands where the lines carefully drawn and habitually held between humanness and wildness begin to dissolve. It is these borderlands where the greatest healing, the strongest magic, the deepest transformation occur.

I want to introduce you to several of the allies I work with most frequently and most deeply. Your relationships with each of them will not be the same as mine, even if you apply their medicine in the same ways that I do, but I hope that my descriptions of the ways I work with each of them and of the nature of their medicine will be of use to you as you begin to develop your own plant relationships.

🌿 Alder (*Alnus* spp.)

Alder grows in liminal places where land and water meet. It shelters Crows and Blackbirds, and Otters make their nests among its roots. In the Welsh tradition, the Alder leaf is the image on the shield of Brân Fendigaidd, a giant king whose name means "Blessed Crow." He made a bridge of his own body for his people to cross, and he brought a cauldron from Wales to Ireland that could bring fallen warriors back to life, a gift to an Irish king who had been wronged by Brân's brother. That same brother broke the peace with that Irish king, resulting in a battle that cost Brân his life. Brân's head is said to be buried beneath the Tower of London and to be the source of the city's protection.

Alder wood was used to make shields throughout Ireland and Britain. The wood is hard and strong, able to resist a blade. When it is cut, it turns blood red. The Irish word for Alder is *fearn,* which is also the name of the Ogham letter with which it is connected. Two phrases describing the meaning of this letter stand out: *airech fian* and *dín cridi.*[1]

Laurie glosses *airech fian* as "shield of warrior bands, vanguard of warrior or hunting bands." As is common with Old Irish, the words have multiple associations. *Airech* as a noun can refer either to a chieftain or to a concubine. *Airech* as an adjective means "careful" or "attentive"—a meaning it retains in modern Irish, though it is now spelled *aireach.*[2] *Fian* refers to a band of warrior poets, outside the jurisdiction of any one ruler, who were defenders of the poor and lived in the forest, an older Irish version of Robin Hood's Merry Men. The word *fian* holds echoes of the name of Fionn MacCumhaill, founder of the first of these warrior bands; *fia,* the word for Deer (and Fionn married a woman who shape-shifted into a deer and together they were the parents of the great poet Ossian); and *fiáin,* the word for wild.

The meaning of *dín cridi* is straightforward and profound. *Dín* means "shelter, protection, defense"; *cridi* means "of the heart."[3] The

Alder grove where I had my vision was a shelter where my heart could open. The cove where I paddle now at twilight most evenings from just after Bealtaine to just after Samhain is a sanctuary where I can transmute what I carry in my heart.

Kiva Rose Hardin, who first introduced me to Alder's medicine, wrote, in a beautiful monograph, that Alder "belongs to the water element, to the deep within where primal transformation takes place."[4] Alder grows in wet places, like the shores of the lake cove where I live, and it nourishes the soil. Hardin describes the relationship between how Alder shifts conditions in the places where it grows and how Alder shifts conditions within the body. She says it is "a remedy deeply aligned with the flow and transformation of fluids in the waterways of the wetland ecologies it grows within as well as the blood and lymph of the human body."[5] Those waters of the body carry the molecular traces of our untransmuted sadness.

When I was sick with COVID-19 just before Bealtaine of 2020, I gathered Alder cones (Alder is one of the few deciduous trees that bears cones) and combined them with Pine cones and boughs to create a steam to help clear the fluid from my lungs that holds old grief. In the months that followed, I gathered Alder catkins and Alder leaves and made a tincture to clear metabolic wastes from my lymph and my blood, to soothe and resolve lingering inflammation. Both applications of Alder I learned from Kiva Rose Hardin. The following spring, I ate Alder catkins fresh from the tree to help resolve the inflammation that was part of my body's healthy response to an mRNA vaccine. I also took Hawthorn and Yarrow for this purpose and drop doses of *Psilocybe cubensis* oxymel, an herbal extraction of honey and vinegar, to aid in immune learning.

Alder is a tree that clears the way for healing and nourishes the life that returns.

Safety considerations: None.
Ecological considerations: Prolific.

🌿 Apple (*Malus* spp.)

The Apple is generous with its sweet fruit, beloved by humans and Bears alike as they prepare for the long months of winter. Like the Bear, the Apple tree goes dormant for the winter.

Part of this is because the Apple is a deciduous tree. But before the leaves of the Apple have all fallen, it has already begun to prepare itself for winter. I learned from Stephen Buhner that as Apples ferment beneath the tree in the autumn sun, their roots drink in the alcohol of their own fruit. As they become drunk on their own cider, the Apples begin to drift into a peaceful sleep. I have often wondered if the British custom of wassailing—pouring cider on the roots of the Apple trees and singing to them as Yuletide ends—might originally be rooted in an understanding that the dreaming of the tree is a kind of gestation that brings fertility in seasons to come and that the gift of cider and song aids in that dreaming.

Perhaps because of the ethereal white of its blossoms in spring and the simultaneously sweet and pungent scent of its fruits fermenting into the soil after they fall to the ground in autumn, the Irish and the Scots and their Welsh and Cornish cousins associated the Apple with the Otherworld. King Arthur (whose name is related to the Welsh and Old Irish words for "bear," *arth* and *arathe*) was famously taken to Avalon, the Island of Apples, when he was grievously wounded in battle, so he could recover and return again in his people's greatest time of need. Manannán mac Lir lives on Emhain Abhlac, which also means the "Island of Apples." The Silver Branch with which he bestows Otherworldly vision on people of this world (see chapter 5) is an Apple branch that bears fruit and blossoms at the same time. The simultaneous fruiting and blossoming mark the branch as coming from a tree that grows in a place outside time.

In Norse tradition, Apples have similar associations. They are connected with the Lady, or the great goddess, and her gift of life. Maria Kvilhaug writes:

The Norse gods, the Aesir, were not immortal. They were completely dependent on the goddess Iðunn, the aspect of the great goddess that offers the apples of eternal resurrection. Every year, they have to eat these apples, and will grow old and die unless she offers these fruits to them. Thus the gods live long through the help of the Lady, but they are not immortal.[6]

Echoes of this association between the Apple and the Lady remained alive in English culture well into the Middle Ages. Remember that while English culture includes elements of Roman culture and of pre-Roman Brythonic Celtic culture, the Saxons were a Scandinavian people who came from Denmark and brought their devotion to the Lady, who they called Freyja, and her twin brother, Freyr, with them over the sea.

The connection of the Apple with the Lady begins, of course, with its fecundity. But it also connected with the fact that when you cut an Apple down the middle, its five seeds form a pentagram. The association of the pentagram with the life-giving aspect of the Lady is attested to as late as the 1400s in the poetic telling of the tale of Sir Gawain and the Green Knight, in which Gawain paints the pentagram on his shield to invoke the Lady's blessing when riding out to meet the seemingly immortal Green Knight.

It is also worth noting that Eve is depicted in European Christian culture as holding an Apple, which is the forbidden fruit of the knowledge of life and death, good and evil. It is far more likely that in its original context, that fruit was a Pomegranate—also associated with fertility and immortality. Some offer linguistic explanations for that transformation, rooted either in confusion about the Latin word *pom,* or in an intentional or unintentional pun on the word *malus,* which as a noun means "Apple" and as an adjective means "malice." Maybe so. But it seems unlikely to be a coincidence that the demonization of the divine feminine in the Middle East was accomplished in a story where a woman corrupts humanity with the fruit associated with the fertility goddesses of that region, and in Europe the symbol shifts to become the fruit associated with the gift of fertility and life from European goddesses.

The twin association with fertility and with the Otherworld made Apples central to a Samhain fortune-telling custom that started in the Scottish Highlands and spread to parts of Ireland, Appalachia, and New England. At Samhain, a girl peels an Apple in a spiraling way, all in one cut, and throws it over her shoulder. The Apple peel will twist into the shape of the initial of her true love to be. A similar custom exists in Chinese culture: a young girl peels an apple while looking in a mirror, and if she does not break the string of peel, the face of her husband will appear in the mirror.

I place Apples on altars to the Lady when making prayers for fertility, healing, or abundance. In winter, I place them outside as an offering to her that will also feed the Deer and the birds during the hungry months.

I also have a special relationship with the feral Apple trees of New England. David Thoreau, who loved the Maine woods where I live, writes: "Our wild apple is wild only like myself, perchance, who belong not to the aboriginal race here, but have strayed into the woods from cultivated stock."[7]

The ancestors of the Apple trees that grow here were brought from Europe and shaped and tended by human hands and human intention to try to produce a uniformly sweet fruit. Over time, some orchards were left untended, and some seeds were spread to wilder places by Bears, Deer, Waxwings, Cardinals, Buntings, and Wrens. Combining their ancestral memory of European forests with their lived experience of the soil, wind, rain, and snow of a very different time and place, they changed. They grew tart fruit that tasted more like the fruit the first people to gather Apples would have known—but also new and different in subtle ways even from the other Crab Apples that grew across the ridge or on the other side of the river.

So the wild Apple is in many ways an emblem of my medicine and my magic. I am neither of the culture around me nor of the culture of my ancestors. What I write here might be less strange to my ancestors than it would be to my neighbors, but it would be new and different to both.

Safety considerations: The seeds can be toxic in large amounts.
Ecological considerations: Abundant.

⚘ Birch (*Betula* spp.)

Praying by firelight close to Imbolc, I had a vision of a king at the center of a circle of women dressed in white, illuminated by starlight. He had just emerged from a season of dreaming in a stone chamber, and they were calling his spirit back into his body and back into the world.

Just before that next Lughnassadh, atop a hill overlooking the Burren, the rocky landscape of western Clare, I saw the vision embodied by a lone Oak growing in the center of a ring of Birches. The Burren was once thick with Oak, Birch, and Hazel before the government of Queen Elizabeth I ordered the cutting of Ireland's forests, which provided sanctuary for rebel bands. In the wake of the destruction of the forest, the soil washed out to the sea. But atop this hill, in a meadow of Heather and Gorse, which I had entered through one of the last intact patches of forest in the area, a lone Oak sapling had grown up under the protection of Birches, and now its crown rose above theirs and sheltered them as they had sheltered it.

Birch is an early succession tree, an opener of the way, creating the conditions that allow forests to return. The Ogham letter *beith,* which is also the first letter of Brighid's name, and the Nordic rune *berkana* are both connected with the tree and with concepts of births, beginnings, and regeneration. Norwegian American Völva, Kari Tauring, writes:

> The Birch was and still is a sacred, goddess, life-line tree in all Northern circumpolar cultures. . . . Ecologically, birch is the tree of regeneration. When the old forest is cleared of hardwoods by lumbering, fire or ice flows, the birch is the first to return. Because of its ability to give birth to a new habitat, the birch is called the mother tree or Nursery tree. It protects the new hard woods until they can take over. When the hard wood takes over and the nursemaid is no

longer needed, they die in place and are called the 'standing dead,' still useful and preserved in their birch bark tombs. When they do fall, they become the undergrowth that the hard woods depend upon to gain their might, height and strength.[8]

In Chernobyl, when people were forced to abandon the region, Birch trees grew up where streets had been, and the Deer and Wolves returned. Chaga mushrooms grew on the bodies of the older Birches—mushrooms whose decoction bears the hint of the taste of Birch and which are known for their capacity to help slow or reverse several types of cancer associated with high radiation levels. The Birch is helping the land regenerate.

In Irish, Scottish, Nordic, Baltic, Slavic, and Germanic traditions, this association with emerging forests, the white color of the tree's bark, the simultaneously soothing and invigorating scent of the leaves and the sap, and the character of their medicine make Birch associated with purification. The best-known connection between the Birch and purifi-cation is its use in the sauna. (We will likely never know if it was used in similar ways in Irish and Scottish sweathouses.) Tauring writes:

> Birch is sacred to the sauna (Finno-Ugric) or pirtz (Baltic) steam bath rituals. Bundles of birch leaves are used to slap the skin to stim-ulate circulation and waken up the senses. There is a runo in Votic (Finno-Ugric), a ritual whisking of the bride and sauna song. There they use three birch twigs and five thin switches before sprinkling the hot rocks with sacred waters."[9]

Birch tea is physiologically cleansing as well. Matthew Wood writes:

> In Germany, it is traditional to use the tea of the leaves of the spring sap of the birch (*Betula alba*) to remove proteinaceous and mineral wastes from the blood, muscles, and joints. The tea of the leaves is a nonirritating diuretic that removes these waste products without inflaming the kidneys.[10]

He also notes that it opens the sweat glands, further helping the body to eliminate waste and making it a perfect medicine for the sweathouse or the sauna. The twigs and the buds can be used for making teas as well. When cutting Birch twigs for medicine in spring, I love the intimacy of drinking the sap that runs from the wound, and the invigorating sense the sap itself brings of life's fecundity and virility.

At Imbolc, I gather fallen Birch branches and strips of fallen Birch bark from the snow to adorn my altar. The bark will often be the centerpiece on which I place my candleholder. Like the lengthening daylight, Birch prepares the way for life's return.

Safety considerations: None.
Ecological considerations: Abundant and prolific.

ꙮ Black Cohosh (*Cimicifuga racemosa*)

Black Cohosh is a plant with dark, gnarled, twisted roots that give rise to a tall stalk topped with a spray of white flowers. It is native to Appalachia and is threatened by overharvesting in its native habitat, so please seek Black Cohosh from growers who cultivate it, or better yet, if you live somewhere where it will thrive, grow it yourself.

Black Cohosh is indicated when someone is in despair, brooding over loss and pain and worry, with grief hanging over them like the proverbial black cloud. There is often tension and a dull ache in the trapezius, a hunched-over posture, and a heavy feeling in the chest. These people will also have a tendency to take on other people's grief.

I think of the spray of white flowers, high above the gnarled root, as the stars that show the way up out of the abyss—or at least are a reminder that there is a world beyond the well. The well of grief can be an important place to spend time. In Irish tradition, all the rivers and streams of the world have their root in a well in the Otherworld beneath our feet—the place of all beginnings and endings. To me, the well of deep grief is that same well, and awash in its waters, we release the meanings the world held before and prepare ourselves to create new meaning as we relate to the world in a new way. But eventually, we need to return to the world. I have found Black Cohosh helps to shift the stagnant emotions that are weighing me down and help me see the starry sky. This reminds me that the iron in my blood and the iron at the core of Earth were forged together in the first generation of stars, that I am connected with everything.

Many contemporary herbalists speak of Black Cohosh as working on estrogen levels through various proposed mechanisms that shift and change as each model becomes outdated. They presume that the depression Black Cohosh treats is associated with estrogen levels, pointing to the greater prevalence of this kind of brooding depression before menstruation, the role of Black Cohosh in easing menstrual pain and in bringing on delayed menstruation, and anecdotal evidence that this kind of depression is most common in women. But I have used Black Cohosh to ease this kind of depression in people of all genders and with all kinds of hormonal profiles. If brooding depression is most prevalent among women, it may be because our society asks women to take on the responsibility for other people's emotions—especially those of men. And Black Cohosh's role in bringing on menstruation can be explained as much through its action on nerves, muscles, fascia, and fluids as it can by a hormonal model of its action.

The great nineteenth-century physio-medicalist physician William Cook saw Black Cohosh acting primarily on nerves and the serous tissues (fascia). Cook began his description of the plant's properties by writing:

> The root of cimicifuga has long been known to American physicians as a remedy of decided and peculiar value; yet its true action has been enshrouded in so much uncertainty that the proper places to employ it have not been well defined. After much experience and careful observation in its use, I offer the following account of it, which I believe to be correct, though in many respects different from the descriptions usually given.[11]

Those words are equally apt today. Black Cohosh tends to be pigeonholed as a women's herb, a menopause herb, or a childbirth herb, when, in fact, these specific uses are just extensions of the plant's broader capacity to work with the nervous system, and by extension, the muscles, to restore fluidity to experience. Cook writes:

> Its power is expended chiefly upon the nervous structures, beginning at the peripheries and extending to the brain, including the ganglionic system; through the sensory nerves influencing the heart and pulse, and through the sympathetic nerves making a decided impression upon the uterus. . . . On the nerves it acts gradually, yet in the end with decided power—soothing them, relieving pain dependent on local irritation, and proving a good antispasmodic.[12]

A well-made Black Cohosh tincture has an earthy taste, like clean soil, with a hint of bitterness—it grounds us in the body. It has a hit of acridity, and the activation of the acrid taste receptor at the back of the throat sends a strong signal across the ventral branch of the vagus nerve, restoring coherent communication between the body's major centers of neurological activity and consciousness (the brain, the heart, the gut, and the genitals) and engaging the parasympathetic nervous system to relax muscular tension throughout the body.

Grounding in the body and improving the flow of communication between our major centers of consciousness makes Black Cohosh an ideal herb for bringing a person into a calm, centered, embodied presence. It is through the heart that we take in the information that forms our emotional felt sense of the world. And it is through the ways in which the enteric portion of our autonomic nervous system reads the signals of tension and flow across the fascia that we gain our visceral sense of the experience of body and world in this location in time and space. Because of this, bringing these centers back into alignment and coherence fundamentally shifts our experience of embodiment. I think of Black Cohosh as realigning a vertical axis of embodied consciousness that also becomes our own axis mundi—the axis on which our world turns. We can extend our awareness along that axis all the way down into the core of Earth, where we can anchor and reorient ourselves and remember who we are.

From this state, we are better able to address and process the grief and pain and fear held in the body. Here, too, Cook's insights guide us to seeing how Black Cohosh can restore the body to healthy flow: "On serous tissues it allays irritation, soothes excitement, and relieves subacute and chronic inflammation."[13]

We can gloss the nineteenth-century use of the term *serous tissue* to refer to what Ida Rolf would call the fascia and stodgy anatomists would call the connective tissues, interstitia, and adipose tissues. The fascia hold our bodies' memories of tension and motion and especially of patterns we have been unable to release. Osteopath Paolo Tozzi discusses this:

> Memories in the body may be also encoded into the structure of fascia itself. Collagen is deposited along the lines of tension imposed or expressed in connective tissues at both molecular and macroscopic level. Mechanical forces acting upon the internal and/or external environment, such as in postures, movements, and strains, dictate the sites where collagen is deposited. Thus, a "tensional memory" is created in a particular connective tissue architecture formed by oriented collagen fibers. This architecture changes accordingly to modification of habitual lines of tension, providing a possible "medium term memory" of the forces imposed on the organism. However, this type of signaling may be altered in pathological conditions. . . . The release of substance P from nerve endings, particularly driven by the hypothalamus following emotional trauma, may alter the collagen structure into a specific hexagonal shape, referred as "emotional scar." The entirety of this phenomenon may be interpreted as a highly structurally and functionally specific process of encoding memory traces in fascia.[14]

Our bodies are mostly water, and the fluids flowing through the collagen bundles of our fascia are a medium of consciousness—carrying hormones and conducting electricity and light, including the biophotons produced by the DNA in the nucleus of every cell. The tissues they flow through are like layers of soil, holding the memory of emotion and sensation. And just as water absorbs the substances contained in layers of soil, so too those inner waters take on the chemical reminders and electromagnetic patterns of the past experiences encoded in the collagen structures. Dancer and occult publisher Alkistis Dimech writes:

> The matrix of connective tissue is the repository of our individual and ancestral memory. (cf. Freud's notion of an "archaic heritage" and Jung's description of archetypes as "biological instinctual constellations.") It is attuned to motion and emotion, which it registers and retains, submerged in and holographically distributed throughout the liquid crystalline continuum. This body memory—which is always oriented to the future, that is, to survival and evolution—is engaged directly through the dynamics of the living body.[15]

Where the body holds patterns of tension and constriction, tissues tend toward low-grade inflammation (creating the dull aches for which Black Cohosh is specific). This creates swelling that further obstructs the flow of fluids, and emotions stagnate—contributing to the kind of dark, heavy, stagnant, brooding emotional state that Black Cohosh is also specific for. My best guess is that Black Cohosh brings down the inflammation in the tissues, allowing the fluids to flow again.

Time and time again I have watched Black Cohosh bring sensory and emotional memories to the surface to be processed and released in ways similar to deep body work. The difference I observe is that Black Cohosh's soothing action on the nervous system usually prevents the surfacing sensations and emotions from becoming too much for the person to bear.

I frequently combine Black Cohosh with Solomon's Seal (*Polygonatum biflorum*) or Shatavari (*Asparagus racemosus*), which lubricate the fascia by promoting the secretion of synovial fluid—and which also make life juicier. Solomon's Seal is threatened in the wild, so please only buy from cultivated sources or grow your own. I will often also bring in a warming aromatic herb to encourage blood flow into—and out of—the tissues, because where blood flows, awareness goes and can shift. Which plant I will use will depend on some of the more esoteric qualities of the plants: I will use Calamus (*Acorus calamus*) if a person needs to bring her emotions and experience into expression, Wormwood (*Artemisia absinthium*) if the person has been beaten down by oppression and feels like the walking dead, Devil's Club (*Oplopanax horridus*) when a person needs to reassert his sense of self and his right to be alive and embodied in the world, and, if things feel physically cold and stuck, Ginger (*Zingiber officinale*)—an idea that comes from a formula of Black Cohosh, Solomon's Seal, and Ginger for joint pain that Margi Flint once taught me and that was my introduction to the energetic pattern underlying all these combinations. Together, these herbs restore flow.

Black Cohosh eases the way for life to flow through us and guides us toward the stars that were the furnaces that forged the elements of our bodies. It is a profound medicine for bringing people into embodied presence.

> **Safety considerations:** large doses may induce labor.
>
> **Ecological considerations:** This plant has become rare in many places due to overharvesting. Obtain it from someone who grows it or someone with impeccable wildcrafting ethics, learn to grow it yourself, or learn to harvest it respectfully from someone with many years of intimate knowledge of the plant's ecology.

❧ Blackthorn (*Prunus spinosa*)

A field in the shadow of Pahto (Mount Adams in Washington), where I once lived, is filled with Blackthorn trees. In autumn, the air echoes with the bugling of rutting Elk. In winter, Elk bones turn up scattered by Coyotes that had come to feed on a carcass likely brought down by a

Mountain Lion. The tallest of the Blackthorns sits alone atop a mound in the center of the field. In the years that I lived there, that tree was the place where I would leave offerings of milk, whiskey, and honey and pray for guidance from the Otherworld.

In springtime, the Blackthorn brings forth bright blossoms before it brings its first leaves. The striking contrast between the white of the flowers and the dark cast of the wood made it a symbol of feminine beauty in Ireland historically. Mac Coitir quotes one early Irish poem that says: *Tá mo ghrá-sa mar bhláth na n-airne ar an draighneán donn* (My love is like the flower on the dark blackthorn).[16]

The black and the white also suggest that beauty has Otherworldly associations. When I made offerings to the Blackthorn in that field, it was the spirit of the land herself who came in shimmering form to receive them. Traditionally, this tree is associated with the *leannán sidhe,* or Faerie lover, a muse who comes to poets and musicians and inspires them to create works of sublime beauty, but who often will inspire a devotion so ardent that the fire in their heads burns too hot for too long and they come to an early death. When engaging a spirit such as this, it is necessary to attend deeply to your body's nourishment and well-being, and to balance engagement with her world with the engaging beauty of this world. I do not believe an early death is a necessary price of such inspiration, but it can be the price of following a vision with such fervor that you neglect your own health and fall out of love with your own body and your own world.

In Ireland, Blackthorn and Hawthorn abound in hedgerows and provide a protective ring around the remaining patches of old forest. Thorny plants tend to fill this ecological role, protecting vulnerable places from intrusion, and they tend to have similar role in the magic and folk traditions of the people of the land where they grow. So it is with Blackthorn. The tree is famously the source of the hard wood of the shillelagh (*saill éalaigh*), a Blackthorn stick seasoned in a chimney above a peat fire for several months and hence turned black by soot, which serves as a club, a walking stick, and a protective charm against magical attacks.

The tree itself is sometimes planted to protect holy places and to hold secrets. Laurie says that in the Ogham alphabet, *straif,* the letter connected with the tree, is associated with the phrase *mórad rún,* "increase of secrets."[17] I learned this aspect of Blackthorn medicine in a fitting way. I was walking through a field in Clare with a group of people I was traveling with and an old fellow from Tipperary. As we passed the Blackthorn, the old fellow said: "I'm not going to talk about the *piseog.* You don't know about the piseog, do you?"

Piseog is an Irish word for a charm or a spell. I told him: "Well, I do know a little bit about the piseog."

He looked surprised and he replied: "Well, I'm not going to tell you about the piseog. If I did I would tell you it was the women who made the piseog, but I am not going to tell you about the piseog. Of course, it's the oldest woman in the family what makes the piseog, but I am not going to tell you about the piseog. She makes it with the egg and the Blackthorn. But I am not going to tell you about the piseog. She makes it with the egg and the Blackthorn. And she plants the Blackthorn, four of them, one in each direction, around the well to protect the well. But I'm not going tell you about the piseog."

I smiled and thought about how very old this custom must be. The matriarch as the guardian of the well, the Blackthorn as her ally. It may well reach back to the Neolithic. Mac Coitir notes that "the overall evidence points to blackthorn being seen as a 'female' tree linked to warlike or fierce female spirits, perhaps derived ultimately from the war goddesses of Pagan Ireland."[18]

The goddess connected with warfare among the Tuath Dé is known as the Morrigan, the Great Queen. Whether she is a single goddess, a trinity of goddesses, or a goddess who wears different names and faces at different times is ambiguous from the old texts. Whether one or three, she is associated with the Ravens and Crows of the battlefield and with prophecy, magic, sovereignty, and warfare. Though it is important to note, as Irish reconstructionist Morgan Daimler does, that war and warriorship in ancient Ireland tended to be ritualized, contained, and governed by codes of honor, as they are in Indigenous cultures around the world. Daimler writes:

> A thoroughly modern problem of the Morrigan as an ancient Irish war Goddess is simply that we, as modern people, often don't understand what war was to the early Irish and hence what exactly a war Goddess was to them. Our modern wars are a far, far cry from the ancient battles and our society is structured in entirely different ways. While war has been and will always be a bloody, dangerous affair, war to the early Irish often revolved around cattle raids and involved small groups rather than huge armies as we would understand that concept today. Battle was done in a strictly honorable way, in equal combat often one-on-one or with matched armies, and we see this emphasized repeatedly in the old stories.[19]

As a goddess of war, the Morrigan would sometimes appear as a foreboding figure warning of coming violence, sometimes as a ritual mourner of the dead, and sometimes would bring favor to warriors she deemed honorable. The most striking and famous example of the latter involved the Morrigan making love in a river to the Dagda, a chieftain among the Tuath Dé, known for his skill in battle, his skill in music, and his generosity of spirit, as the Tuath Dé prepared for their war against the Fomorians, who had enslaved and impoverished the other peoples of Ireland and brought ruin to the land. After the Morrigan took the Dagda as her lover, the Tuath Dé were blessed with luck and valor and the Fomorians were cursed with weakness and misfortune.

It was in the time just before Samhain that the Morrigan and the Dagda came together—the fierce woman who protected the land and the generous chieftain whose cauldron fed the people and the land. Their coming together blessed the land with fertility in the seasons to come. This is one of the oldest initiations of a sacral king in Ireland, and in many ways it was this act that was replayed in the wedding of the rí to the land in November. In the old epic tale of the war between the Tuath Dé and the Fomorians, the passage that recounts their wedding refers to her as "the Morrigan, whose name was Anand." This may link her to Anu, considered to be the mother of the Tuath Dé, and possibly to Áine, the sovereignty goddess of the province of Munster. Though these connections are impossible to prove or disprove on a purely textual or historical basis, they are things that can be understood only through relating with the spirits who bear these names.

But there is another significant echo in the name Anand—its similarity to *ananda,* the Sanskrit word for "bliss." Irish is an Indo-European language with roots in common with Sanskrit, and this echo seems too close to be mere coincidence, especially when referring to the Morrigan appearing as holy lover to a righteous warrior. These two aspects of her being—pleasure and ferocity, beauty and terror—are not contradictory and are also present in the Blackthorn.

While the wood of the Blackthorn has a martial and protective nature, the flower and the leaf, like those of the Blackthorn's botanical sisters, Peach and Cherry, have a soothing medicine that cools inflammation and calms the mind. A student in Spain tells me that the leaves are traditionally smoked there as a gentle sedative. I am not aware of any similar tradition being extant in Ireland, but Laurie does mention the association of the Ogham letter *straif* with the phrase *saigid nél,* literally "seeking of clouds," which refers to divination in the shapes made by smoke. For one Samhain I mixed dried Blackthorn leaves with Mugwort to make an incense for divination. Breathing in the smoke, of course, relaxes the mind and makes it receptive.

The berry of the Blackthorn is called the sloe in English and the *airne* in Irish—source of the name of my ancestral home, Killarney or Cuille Airne, Church of the Sloes. The berry was traditionally fermented to make a wine drunk at Samhain in some parts of Ireland. Modern people are more likely to have encountered it as one of the flavorings in sloe gin, where, interestingly, it is paired with Juniper, a traditional Scottish herb of blessing and purification.

Safety considerations: None.

Ecological considerations: Abundant in its traditional European homeland and invasive in the areas where it has become naturalized in North America.

🌿 Calamus (*Acorus calamus*)

In Chinese medicine, the heart is the primary organ of consciousness and perception. The watery heart yin represents the heart's capacity to take in information from the world: it is nourished by beauty. The senses are spoken of as the "orifices of the heart." The fiery heart yang represents our capacity to express ourselves.

When we are overwhelmed with sensory and emotional information, the heart yin can overwhelm the heart yang, clouding the senses with a fog and first obscuring and then drowning out the fire of expression. Think of the heavy, dull feeling that lingers in your head after being in a noisy, crowded store with bright fluorescent lights in December. Intense memories—sensation and emotion reexperienced outside their original context—bring their own fog, cutting us off from the experience of being present here and now. They can distort our perception of current events and prevent us from responding coherently.

Growing in the marshy muck of the shallows of lakes and ponds, Calamus, with its green rush-like leaves and its bright yellow or green spathe, has a spicy root that clears the waters of the heart by reigniting the heart yang. Its sweet scent engages the senses, its bitterness grounds us and activates the enteric nervous system that processes the sensory information coming in from the fascia of the entire body, and its pungent heat focuses the mind and senses and stimulates circulation to the brain.

This makes it an especially important medicine for Autistic people like me. Sensory gating is the process by which people filter sensory information—including the felt sense of others' emotions and our own—so we only have to consciously interpret the information that is most important and most relevant, parameters set both by our belief structures and our bodies' past experiences. The sensory gating channels of Autistic people tend to be more wide open than most people, which allows them to perceive things others miss but can also overwhelm them with information that they have a hard time prioritizing and sorting. In response, Autistic people can go into sensory shutdown, and those who usually have access to speech can lose that access altogether.

When this happens to me, a few minutes in a dark room and a few drops of Calamus can often help me reorient and recover my ability to speak. Hawthorn is often a nice addition to the Calamus, helping to soothe the hyperreactivity of my senses by cooling the heart (and possibly by reducing histamine and other proinflammatory compounds in my blood vessels). Schisandra can be a nice addition as well, helping to gather my attention inward toward my heart.

This dovetails with another capacity of Calamus—the capacity to refine perception and expression. Ayurveda, which shares ancient cultural roots with Irish tradition going back to the Neolithic, speaks of kundalini, the vital force, likened to a rising serpent, that flows from its genital root up the spine to the head. Ancient Greek and Middle Eastern traditions similarly spoke of twin serpents that climb the spine and are instruments of the fluid transmission of consciousness that leaves the body at death. Ayurveda describes Calamus—which it calls *vacha,* a Sanskrit word for "voice"—as an herb that purifies the kundalini to bring clear perception and understanding. It also has a long history of use in incense and anointing oils in Egypt and in much of the Middle East.

Calamus is not just an herb that aids in bringing forth speech; it also aids in bringing forth the heart's purest truth. Herbalist jim mcdonald, who first introduced me to this herb, speaks of it as an herb that can help people who have plateaued in their mental and emotional processing of their lives to achieve new insights, and I have seen Calamus do this again and again.

This is also an herb I give to people when they need the courage and clarity to speak difficult truths. If it had a motto, it might be that of the late Maggie Kuhn, founder of the Gray Panthers, who implored people: "Speak your mind—even if your voice shakes."[20]

Safety considerations: Rodent studies of high intravenous doses of one isolated constituent of Calamus showed liver damage in the test subjects. I personally feel very safe with small to moderate doses of the plant. The plant does accumulate toxins from soil, so be careful where you grow or harvest it.

Ecological considerations: Prolific in some areas in the wild and fairly easily cultivated.

Cannabis (*Cannabis indica* and *Cannabis sativa*)

The human relationship with Cannabis is long and complex. Humans began growing Cannabis early in the history of agricultural civilization, but the first archaeological evidence of its ritual use shows up in burials in Central Asia around 500 BCE and in the Middle East around three centuries later.[21] Greek sources make reference to Scythian and Thracian ritual uses of the plant in the first century of the Common Era. In India, some sects hold the plant to be sacred to the god Shiva.[22] Ritual use of the plant had spread to North Africa by the end of the first millennium,[23] but there is no evidence to support popular claims that the plant played a role in European witchcraft in the medieval or Early Modern periods. Rural European rituals of that era favored nightshades and Artemesias as consciousness-altering ointments and smokes.

Medical use of Cannabis is documented in first-century Chinese texts. It was primarily used in this era as a remedy for constipation, rheumatic pain, malaria, and menstrual disorders or as an analgesic during surgery. However, one intriguing passage in the oldest printed Chinese pharmacopeia warns that excess consumption of the plant can cause one to see devils in the short term and over the long term can impart the ability to communicate with spirits and a "lightness" of being.[24]

This openness to spirit communication, for good and for ill, is a hallmark of shamanic and magical understandings of Cannabis across history. For those adept at communicating with spirits, Cannabis can be a facilitator of that communication. However, not all disembodied spirits have our best interests in mind, and not all people are well suited to opening up their connection with the spirit realm.

Cannabis made its appearance in North American and Western European culture as a medicine and a drug of consciousness alteration in the nineteenth century, arriving initially from the Middle East and India.[25] The great eclectic physician Finley Ellingwood described the plant as an anodyne, sedative, and antispasmodic with particular relevance to disorders of the nervous system, the reproductive-generative system, and the urinary tract.[26] In homeopathic dilutions, it was used primarily for bladder infections and is still used this way today.[27] The use of the plant as a urinary tract antispasmodic is largely forgotten today in herbal medicine—ironic in an era where proponents suggest Cannabis as a panacea. I have seen it work wonders in reversing temporary urinary paralysis caused by stress or by overuse of ketamine. For these purposes, I combine it with Kava (*Piper methysticum*) and Mullein root (*Verbascum* spp.)

In the twentieth century, artistic and cultural movements associated first with jazz, then with rock and roll, and then with hip-hop, occurring roughly at thirty-year intervals, popularized the recreational use of Cannabis in North America and Europe. Backlash against the 1960s counterculture led to the now discredited idea that Cannabis is a "gateway drug." As so often occurs, however, the distortion points to a hidden truth: for many people, Cannabis is a gateway plant—the first plant they experience as noticeably shifting their consciousness and of possessing a consciousness of its own.

Medicinal Cannabis reached new prominence in the 1980s and the 1990s largely as a result of the work of people in the Queer community in San Francisco who began using the plant to treat pain and wasting syndromes associated with HIV/AIDS and advocating for access to the medicine for those who needed it.[28]

Research into Cannabis pharmacology revealed that the plant has a large number of unique fat-soluble phenolic compounds collectively known as cannabinoids. The search for the mechanism of action of these compounds led to the discovery of a new system within the body: the endocannabinoid system. More on that in a moment.

THC and cannabidiol (CBD) are the two most well-known of the cannabinoids. The level of THC present in a Cannabis plant determines whether it is legally considered Marijuana or Hemp. In the United States, Cannabis plants with less than 0.3 percent THC by volume are designated as Hemp and are legal in all states and in interstate commerce. Cannabis plants with higher THC content are legal in most states for medical purposes and in several states for any use by adults but are illegal in interstate commerce.

THC content and strain genealogies also dictate the botanically specious designation of some Marijuana as *sativa,* some as *indica,* and some as hybrid. *Cannabis indica* and *Cannabis sativa* were initially distinct species, but all Cannabis in commerce in North America is a hybrid of the two strains. The terms *indica* and *sativa* have taken on new cultural and commercial meanings. *Sativa* is commonly used to refer to more mind-altering, emerging strains that generally have higher THC content; *indica* is generally used to refer to more relaxing, sedating strains that usually (but not always) have lower THC content; and hybrids are strains developed by growers who cross strains thought of as *sativas* with those thought of as *indicas.* Ironically, it was originally hemp with low THC levels that was classified as *Cannabis sativa.* One must, therefore, consider the date of literature in assessing references to *indica* or *sativa.*

Now that we have straightened out the legal and commercial taxonomy, let's look at the pharmacology. The nervous system, the immune system, and the endocrine system all work together to coordinate the body's responses to the world. These three body systems are all strongly influenced by the endocannabinoid system—the system of receptor sites in our bodies that respond both to chemicals from the Cannabis plant and to similar compounds we manufacture ourselves. All of the major types of cells involved in inflammation contain endocannabinoids and endocannabinoid receptors, suggesting that the system, when it is healthy, helps keep inflammation in balance.[29]

The endocannabinoid system has two primary sets of receptors: CB-1 receptors and CB-2 receptors. CB-1 receptors are present primarily in the central nervous system where they help regulate brain activity. Phytocannabinoids (cannabinoids from plants) and endocannabinoids have a unique way of acting on the nervous system: reverse signaling. They essentially allow individual neurons to talk back to the rest of the nervous system, signaling the neuron that would normally come before them in the signaling chain to either tamp down or increase the release of neurotransmitters from one neuron to another. (This is an oversimplification that I will let stand for the moment.)

CB-2 receptors are widely distributed throughout the body but largely absent in the central nervous system, except in the microglia, specialized immune cells present in the brain.[30] Microglial inflammation may contribute to degenerative neurological diseases, and stimulation of the CB-2 receptors in the microglia may have a protective effect.[31] Some forms of depression may be caused by microglial inflammation, and it is interesting in this regard to note that Ellingwood spoke of Cannabis as a remedy in melancholia and in meningitis.[32] Might reduction of microglial inflammation be an operative factor in both uses?

The endocannabinoid system extends into the hypothalamus and can essentially put the brakes on the HPA axis, regulating our stress response.[33] Our own body creates molecules similar to the ones in the Cannabis plant to help manage stress.[34] One of the most important of these compounds is anandamide. *Ananda*, as we learned earlier, is the Sanskrit word for bliss. True to its name, anandamide helps us experience pleasure. It also exerts a positive influence on the entire endocannabinoid system. The presence of anandamide precursors and analogs in Cacao may partially explain why so many people enjoy chocolate.[35]

Through modulating neurological, endocrine, and immune function in the tissues where they are present, endocannabinoids are complex regulatory molecules that can modulate almost any function in the body. Some researchers theorize that an endocannabinoid deficiency may play a role in chronic pain and inflammation in diseases like

170 Plant and Fungal Allies

fibromyalgia and irritable bowel syndrome and possibly even depression. Ethan Russo points out the role that endocannabinoids play in regulating mood and digestion and reducing pain and suggests that "if endocannabinoid function were decreased, it follows that a lowered pain threshold would be operative, along with derangements of digestion, mood, and sleep among the almost universal physiological systems subserved by the endocannabinoid system."[36]

There are two important caveats when considering Russo's point. The first is that endocannabinoid deficiency is likely a marker or symptom of a larger dysregulation; the root causes of which, from the holistic standpoint, must ultimately be addressed. Alcohol, stress, and sleep deprivation also impair function of the endocannabinoid system. The second is that there are ways other than, or in addition to, working with Marijuana and Hemp to support endocannabinoid system health. Physician Dustin Sulak notes that "a diet high in Omega-3 and low in Omega-6 fatty acids supports healthy function of the endocannabinoid system."[37] In addition to Cacao (*Theobroma cacao*), Turmeric (*Curcuma* spp.) and Tea (*Camellia sinensis*) appear to act on the endocannabinoid system as a whole, and Echinacea (*Echinacea* spp.) acts on the CB-2 receptors.

All cannabinoids are lipid soluble and can be extracted through the making of an infused oil. As we will see below, however, in order for THC to pass through the blood-brain barrier, it is necessary to further add heat. Chinese herbalism traditionally uses the mechanically extracted oil of Cannabis seeds, which like Flax seeds are rich in polyunsaturated fatty acids, to treat constipation.[38]

Now let's take a look at CBD and THC. In an earlier paper, Russo notes that while we have found many molecules that act on the endocannabinoid system, the "first clinically available" compound that acts to balance the whole system, to modulate the modulators, is CBD.[39] It helps the body use anandamide more efficiently, exerting a modulating influence on both CB-1 and CB-2 receptors and on the HPA axis.[40] For this reason it acts as a general neuro-endocrine-immune modulator.

CBD also has pain-relieving properties. It both directly reduces pain and changes the way the body perceives pain, thereby making it less overwhelming.[41] Research in the past decade has also shown that CBD has strong anxiolytic or antianxiety effects. One way that scientists study anxiety is by getting people to do something that makes most people nervous, such as public speaking. Researchers in Brazil randomly divided people dealing with social anxiety into two groups—one group received CBD and another group received a placebo. Both groups were then given two minutes to prepare a four-minute speech about public transportation. They then had to deliver the speech on camera while watching themselves on a TV screen. The group that received the CBD reported less anxiety, displayed clearer thinking, and felt better about their speeches and about themselves than the people in the group that received the placebo.[42]

Brain scans show that CBD decreases blood flow to the limbic and paralimbic regions, reducing fear and anxiety, preventing the body from going into high alert or helping it calm back down.[43] This may also increase the intensity and salience of other sensations and emotions.

CBD also shows promise in the treatment of PTSD. Our bodies evolved to remember everything about painful and scary situations, so that we can avoid repeating them—this kind of memory is called aversive memory. This is a helpful mechanism in some ways, but it can cause problems too. When we experience something truly horrible, our aversive memories can become so strong and so easily triggered that they can make it hard to function. CBD has the amazing ability to change the ways we create and recall painful memories. It reduces fear as we feel it, prevents the fear from consolidating into memory, helps us to forget the fear and to reduce the nightmares old fears cause, and is gentle enough for children.[44] CBD also shows promise in the treatment of addictions because of its capacity to reduce both the salience of traumatic memories and the salience of the memory of the pleasure received from the substance or activity to which a person is addicted.[45]

THC acts on both CB-1 receptors in the central nervous system and CB-2 receptors throughout the body. Its action on CB-2 receptors tends to complement the action of CBD, modulating inflammation. Its action on CB-1 receptors tends to move things in a different direction than CBD does. Where CBD tends to decrease the salience of stimuli and memories, THC tends to increase their salience both through its direct action on the brain and through facilitating greater dopamine release in the frontal cortex.[46] This can be a blessing or a curse, depending on the person and the situation. As I explained earlier, people who have a tendency toward psychosis or mania can have those tendencies activated or exacerbated by THC, and people who have a tendency toward dopamine-related addictions can develop a dependency on THC.

On the other hand, this dopaminergic action and the increase of the salience of sensations and memories makes this compound a highly pleasurable one for many people and is one of the reasons many people find that Cannabis enhances their creativity. The dopaminergic action of Cannabis can be further potentiated by Damiana and Lobelia. When I work with artists who find themselves feeling creative when working with Cannabis but unable to translate that creativity into productivity, I often have them add a pinch of Mugwort (*Artemesia vulgaris*).

When it comes to anxiety, this can cut both ways. For many people, increasing the dopamine levels increases the amount of dopamine that is available to be converted to norepinephrine and so can lead to fear and paranoia. For others, especially for some but not all Autistic people, increasing the salience of the sensory data coming in can make that data more manageable, and hence THC can relieve anxiety.

THC's stimulation of the CB-1 receptor also plays a role in making people hungry. This is why people get "the munchies." This also makes THC an important compound in helping people with advanced cases of diseases like cancer and HIV/AIDS recover their appetites. Cannabis edibles, of course, can simultaneously cause and address "the munchies." They first entered the popular imagination via a recipe for "Hashcich [sic] Fudge" that Alice B. Toklas, the partner of poet and artist Gertrude Stein, shared in her 1954 cookbook. It is not clear whether Toklas herself ever prepared the recipe; she got it from another artist,

Brion Grysin, who sent it in response to her desperate plea to friends for recipes as the deadline of the cookbook approached.[47] From there it filtered first into beatnik circles and then into hippie circles, becoming the famous pot brownies of the 1970s. Simply baking Cannabis in a recipe that included some fat will extract an appreciable amount of THC, though we will see below that more precision increases the extraction. One peril of Cannabis edibles is that because the THC enters the bloodstream via the digestive tract rather than via the lungs, there is a delayed onset, which can make it difficult for people to gauge how much THC is entering their systems.

Because CB-1 receptors are primarily located in the brain, THC needs to cross the blood-brain barrier to be effective. In raw Cannabis, THC is present in an acidic form, THCA, that cannot pass through that barrier effectively. Though with a large enough exposure to THCA some THC does reach the brain, just ask anyone who has ever trimmed Cannabis about the trancey state they experience from transdermal absorption of THCA. This can be rectified by using heat to break the carboxyl group off the molecule either by smoking or vaporizing the plant or by heating it in an oven before extracting it in oil: remember, cannabinoids are lipophilic, so oil extraction works best. I personally heat it at about 225° F for about 45 minutes and favor Coconut oil. Decarboxylation can also be achieved through smoking or vaporizing Cannabis.

THC can often be more effective in treating neurological pain than CBD alone. One reason is that it appears to alter functional brain connectivity in ways that change how the brain is processing pain signals.[48] Psilocybin works with pain in similar ways. Both are changing the meaning of the sensations. THC is also a potently antispasmodic compound, helping to release tension whether administered topically or internally, and for some it can play an important role in the management of seizures.

All of this talk about individual constituents, however, is ultimately a crude and imprecise shorthand for offering a rationalist explanation of how this plant interacts with us. To presume that one understands

Cannabis just because one has a knowledge of the properties of two constituents would be like presuming to speak a language after learning a handful of words. As with all plants, Cannabis is best understood experientially and relationally, something that is being lost with the commercialization of the plant and that we need to restore to find right relationship with this generous ally.

> **Safety considerations:** Those with a predisposition to manic or psychotic episodes should be careful with this plant. The dopaminergic action of THC can trigger mania or psychosis in people with underlying tendencies toward such conditions.
>
> **Ecological considerations:** Widely cultivated.

🌸 Damiana (*Turnera diffusa*)

Damiana is a light at the southwestern horizon reminding us that, though the night descending is dark, morning will come. Bitter, warming, and aromatic, Damiana grounds us into our bodies, stirs our heart to quicken the rhythm of the movement of our blood, gently opens the airways, and relaxes the tension we hold to allow the blood to flow freely to all of our parts—and where blood flows, awareness goes. Damiana is the one plant I speak of here that I have not come to know in person, but it is a plant so integral to my practice that I would be remiss not to speak of its medicine and magic.

In winters of snow and ice, winters of the heart, and winters of our collective experience, Damiana awakens the memory of the invincible summer within us that Albert Camus spoke of finding in the depths of winter. Damiana is well known for its capacity to stimulate pelvic circulation, bringing blood and awareness flowing to the genitals, giving rise to its reputation as an aphrodisiac. And it excels in this manner.

But to fully appreciate the stirring Damiana brings to the body, we need to broaden our definition of the erotic. Eros is the force that sets matter dancing, the embodied flow of life. By relaxing tension and increasing blood flow and sensation, Damiana invites us to inhabit our bodies more deeply, engaging eros in new ways. It is an herb of joyful embodiment, restoring sensual pleasure in all of its forms—dancing, touching, savoring delicious food, breathing in the scent of snow and Fir and Pine and woodsmoke.

I often give Damiana to elders who are living in a world that forgets that bodies of all ages need and desire sensual pleasure and to people recovering from injuries and illnesses who are learning to be in their bodies again. I sometimes combine Damiana with the Chinese herb *Corydalis yahushua*, usually used to diminish the intensity of pain signals to keep the return of sensation from being too overwhelming at first. Damiana is also delicious in honey and amazing in mead.

Like all bitter, warming aromatic herbs, Damiana is a carminative, stimulating sluggish digestion and relieving gas and bloating. The latter action of carminatives is an important consideration in timing the administration of Damiana as an aphrodisiac in the conventional sense. Damiana has been shown to increase the efficiency of mitochondria— the symbiotic creatures who live within our cells and serve as their metabolic furnaces. The boost in energy and circulation that Damiana brings increases pleasure in movement.

As I mentioned above in our discussion of Lobelia, Damiana also has an important relationship with dopamine. Dopamine and the manipulation of dopamine levels are a hot cultural topic right now, given dopamine's connection with feelings of pleasure and our culture's complex relationship with those feelings. As most conversations about neurotransmitters are, the current popular conversation about dopamine is a bit misleading. Yes, we receive dopamine releases from social media likes, and indeed this is a deliberately engineered phenomenon. It is also true that most substances and activities that people become addicted to stimulate some level of dopamine release, with diminishing returns over time. This has led to the popularity of "dopamine fasts," times of limiting sensory input as a means of self-discipline, and the accompanying idea that we are a society that relies too much on dopamine. But I think we are dealing with a society that in general is in a state of dopamine deficiency rather than dopamine excess. Dopamine is depleted in the manufacture of norepinephrine, and the stress of modern life puts most people in a high norepinephrine state throughout long stretches of their days, and they then crash, and from that depleted place anything that will bring a little dopamine release will be a way out of the gray void for a moment.

But let's zoom out a bit and look at the bigger picture. Dr. Kenneth Proefrock describes dopamine as a molecule that helps to create and reinforce meaning. We get the strongest dopamine (and serotonin) releases from novel, meaningful experiences. In this way, addiction can, in many ways, be thought of as a disease or consequence of a life lacking in meaning. The person is driven to find fleeting meaning in whatever can bring relief or pleasure in the moment. (And I believe everyone is, for the most part, doing the best they can, with the information and resources they have at their disposal, to make their lives meaningful.)

Damiana is a selective MAO-B inhibitor. MAO-A and MAO-B (MAO stands for monoamine oxidase) are the primary enzymes that break down our neurotransmitters. So MAO inhibitors tend to make neurotransmitters stay around for longer. MAO-A breaks down all of our neurotransmitters, so MAO-A inhibitors and broad-spectrum MAO inhibitors like the harmaline in Syrian Rue (*Peganum harmala*) will slow the breakdown of all neurotransmitters—which, yes, means more serotonin and dopamine but also means more norepinephrine and tyramine, which can result in big blood pressure spikes. MAO-B only breaks down dopamine and phenylethylamine. So in inhibiting MAO-B, Damiana helps dopamine stick around for longer, which, when combined with its increase in circulation throughout the body and its sensitization of sensory nerves, makes it feel good to have a body and especially to move and engage a body. It is a heightener of sensory meaning.

Two other herbs that affect these neurotransmitters are Bacopa (*Bacopa monnieri*) and Lobelia. Bacopa contains the dopamine precursor L-Dopa. For L-Dopa to stick around long enough to be made into new dopamine, you need an MAO-inhibitor, and an MAO-B inhibitor will be best for the reasons I described above. As for Bacopa itself, in India it is known as Brahmi, a name that refers to Brahma, a god of creation and destruction. Brahmi is one of the sattvic herbs, meaning it enhances understanding; it is a maker of spiritual and intellectual meaning. Lobelia slows the conversion of dopamine to norepinephrine and activates the parasympathetic nervous system, increasing receptivity to experience and lowering norepinephrine and adrenaline. It is a preserver of meaning.

Take Damiana, Bacopa, and Lobelia together and spend a few hours on social media, and you will likely deepen your addiction to social media. But take these herbs together and engage in something meaningful—such as working out, singing, dancing, reading poetry aloud, performing a simple ritual, working in the garden, walking in the woods, meditating, or praying—and you will get positive reinforcement, even if initially you didn't feel like doing any of those things. So I tend to link dosing with these herbs with practices that deepen meaning.

Safety considerations: Those with personal or family histories of psychosis should use with caution.

Ecological considerations: Overharvested in the wild, seek cultivated source.

▓ Eastern Skunk Cabbage (*Symplocarpus foetidus*)

Eastern Skunk Cabbage is the first plant to poke its head through the ground in the swamps of New England, budding just before Bears come out of their dens. It melts the ice and snow around it by generating heat through a chemical process remarkably similar to that used by hibernating animals to raise their temperature as they rouse from sleep. Depending on how many acorns are left on the ground, Eastern Skunk Cabbage will make up somewhere between 50 percent and 99 percent of a Black Bear's diet in New England in early spring.

Skunk Cabbage is perhaps best known as a respiratory medicine. The 1898 edition of *King's American Dispensatory* describes Eastern Skunk Cabbage root as "a stimulant, exerting expectorant."[49] Just as the plant's contractile roots reach deep into swampy soils to drink up moisture, the root as a medicine brings up excess mucous from deep in the lungs. It is one of only two medicines that I have observed bringing relief to people experiencing the terrifying and so far unexplained bouts of "air hunger" associated with chronic Lyme disease and chronic COVID-19 infection. In air hunger, a person feels unable to breathe in sufficient air and so engages in deep, rapid, and labored breathing. The other medicine that helps here is its cousin, Wester Skunk Cabbage (*Lysichiton americanus*), which Stephen Harrod Buhner first recommended for this symptom.[50]

It has other ways of addressing what we hold deep below as well. Eastern Skunk Cabbage contains 5-hydroxytryptamine, identical to the neurotransmitter serotonin, which is responsible for opening sensory gating channels and encouraging synaptic branching in human nervous systems. At low doses, the tincture of the root induces a deep sense of stillness and calm, like the waters of a vernal pool. William Cook described it as "a simple and reliable nervine, of the most innocent and effective soothing character."[51] At higher doses, the tincture begins to have an entheogenic effect. The world becomes more fluid. Distinctions between thought and emotion dissolve. Tryptamines work to reorder the ways in which we process the information we get from the world. As entheogens, both Eastern Skunk Cabbage (*Symplocarpus foetidus*) and Western Skunk Cabbage (*Lysichiton americanus*) seem to work with the integration of the rational consciousness of the brain and the emotional and transpersonal consciousness of the heart. It's not clear whether Western Skunk Cabbage contains tryptamines, but Stephen Harrod Buhner first observed this phenomenon with a snuff made from Western Skunk Cabbage roots,[52] and I've observed similar effects with the tincture.

Eastern Skunk Cabbage has a strong affinity with the lungs (contemporary and traditional use as a stimulating expectorant), the heart (it is used for a "weak heart" among the Menominee people of the land now called Wisconsin, according to a friend who is part of that culture), and the kidneys and uterus because of its harmony with the waters that flow through our bodies. Thus, at commonly used medicinal doses,

Eastern Skunk Cabbage will help to clear the physical manifestations of grief that gets buried in the lungs.

At large doses in the proper extraction, it begins to address such grief at a soul level through reconnection to the dreaming mind of Earth—especially when potentiated by an MAO-A inhibitor such as Syrian Rue. (Note that MAO-A inhibitors can be dangerous for those with hypertension and those on psychiatric medications.) In the process, it carries a person through the grief of many lifetimes—a harrowing journey, to say the least. Like psilocybin, the serotonin in Skunk Cabbage and the harmaline in Syrian Rue are best extracted in a gently acidic menstruum, like vinegar. In both cases, the healing work is not to be undertaken lightly. The pain released needs a container, and the journey back to the self is a journey through a world fraught with its own perils and challenges. Ecstatic methods require focus to avoid becoming purely chaotic and unleashing unintended consequences.

Eastern Skunk Cabbage can be a vehicle for traveling beneath the surface of the waters of consciousness to encounter the source of the wound and move through it and past it, undoing its power to shape consciousness and define identity. The perils lie in the potential of becoming so immersed in the pain and grief that the journey is never completed. But when the journey is completed, the wound is transformed from a source of pain to an opening between worlds that initiates the traveler into the compassion that comes from understanding grief and into the wellspring of healing. This wellspring lies beneath the surface; it comes from the heart of the universe and rises from the center of our heart to flow outward, blessing and transforming all worlds. Eastern Skunk Cabbage can offer an opening to the realms where such transformation is possible.

This Bear medicine stirs the sleeping Animal Self, awakening us into fuller presence.

Safety considerations: The calcium oxalate crystals in the root can be irritating to both the airways and the digestive tract. A long drying period will reduce their concentration, and they will not extract in a tincturing process. They can be released into the air by chopping the root, so only process the roots in a well-ventilated area while wearing a mask or respirator.

Ecological considerations: While locally abundant in many places, this plant cannot be cultivated, and individual plants can be over a thousand years old, so be very sparing with your harvest. The root of one plant, dug in winter when the plant is first melting through the ice, will produce enough tincture to serve one herbalist for many seasons. And the process of digging and pulling in water and mud just one or two degrees above freezing is quite the initiation into deep relation with this plant. For most, it will be better to make a flower essence: wait until the plant is flowering, and during a new moon or a full moon, place a bowl of water at its base overnight. Gather the water the next morning and mix with an equal part whiskey, poteen, a liquor made from potatoes, or moonshine, made from corn, to preserve it.

🌿 Elecampane (*Inula helenium*)

Grief is a watery thing that works its way into the lungs, moving downward. When the waters become stagnant, infection can set in.

Since early childhood, I have struggled with asthma and frequent bouts of bronchitis, born of grief breathed in and pushed down deep. My great-grandmother died on Christmas Eve when I was five months old. She had a long history of having breathing problems when she became emotional. And she also had a long history of drinking—perhaps to dull her senses. She was a psychically sensitive, college-educated widow living in conservative suburban upstate New York. Her mother's people came to Wisconsin from County Roscommon during the Great Hunger, and from her mother, she inherited the sight. I shared a strange bond with her. I was supposed to meet her the day she died, but I had bronchitis, so my mother did not take me to see her. Months later, my mother saw her ghost move my crib across the bedroom.

I inherited her patterns of breathing. I stuffed down grief and let it fill my lungs until I could not breathe. When it overflowed, I would swallow it and experience horrible gas and indigestion. When it got bad enough, I would throw up, which allowed me to breathe again.

Sensitive to the world, I worried from an early age about endangered species and nuclear war. I was a melancholy, Otherworldly child and a depressed teenager. I felt like I lived in a drowning world and could only pull more of its water into my lungs. My interpretation of Catholic theology, one quite independent of the interpretation I was taught, led me to believe that by taking that grief into myself I could somehow transmute it. The struggle for breath coupled with that theology served to alienate me from my body. And as an adult, I made a profession of being a carrier of other people's stories of suffering.

To recap a story I tell in the introduction to this book: in December of 2005, a few weeks after returning from gathering stories of torture, displacement, and the loss of land and culture in Oaxaca in the south of Mexico, I developed severe bronchitis that had me bedridden on New Year's Eve. A chance phone call that day from a perceptive herbalist I had met at a party the night I returned from Oaxaca resulted in my introduction to Elecampane—a medicine that reaches deep into the lungs and gets things moving again, releasing and cleansing buried grief, just as it brings up old, infected mucus. Matthew Wood writes:

Elecampane is a warming, stimulant, pungent, aromatic bitter that permeates the bronchial tree. It resolves bacterial infection, reducing heavy, thick, green mucus down to yellow and eventually to white or clear mucus. It is specific to yellow and green mucus, indicating bacterial infection. The removal of the layer of old, adhesive mucus allows for the secretion of a new layer of thin, clear mucus that is impregnated with immune factors. Meanwhile, the bitters protect the stomach against indigestion caused by mucus that is swallowed. Very typically, the person needing elecampane (often a child) swallows the mucus.[53]

Wood, of course, is describing—word for word—the pattern of disease I had developed.

I still remember the warm zing of the first drops of Elecampane tincture on my tongue that winter. The day after I started taking Elecampane, I was breathing well enough to take my dog on a long hike through the Bangor City Forest—the very place where, six months later, the *Usnea* lichen would begin to speak to me, claiming me as its own, bringing me deeper into relationship with the wild and beginning to lead me on the path of becoming an herbalist in my own right. Elecampane gave me my breath, and my breath brought me into my body, allowing me to begin to move and transform it, coming into the world in a new way.

Elecampane takes both its common name and its Latin name (*Inula helenium*) from the legend of Helen of Troy. Wood writes: "The legend is that when Helen was kidnapped by Paris, the plant sprang up from where her tears fell. Afterward the plant was known as 'Heart of the Campagna'—elecampane." Wood notes that the plant is indicated for people who have been "torn away from [their] home, causing grief and suffering."[54] I believe that the plant is also often indicated for those who have never felt at home in their surroundings to begin with.

It is a familiar archetype: the bookish, asthmatic child whose imagination is captivated by stories of other worlds that sound more like home than this one. This child is at once distant and emotionally sensitive, at times deeply empathetic and perceptive and at other times completely oblivious to social norms and cues. Asthma, in these cases, is often closely associated with social anxiety. Breath is a tenuous thread barely keeping the child present in this reality. In another time and place, such a child might be called *fae*—perhaps a changeling, a Faerie child left in place of a stolen human one. And indeed, Elecampane is a plant strongly associated with the Faerie realm. In England, it was once commonly known as Elf Dock.

Such feelings of being born into the wrong world and the wrong body can linger into adulthood. And by the time such a child has become an adult, they have often internalized a lifetime of stories about being broken, powerless, and insufficient, eroding confidence. This can lead to an attempt to deny and suppress the sensitivity and vision that are the core of such a person's identity. More emotion pushed down into the lungs, continuing the pattern of illness. This may suggest the plant's possible historical use to treat elf-shot, which Wood describes as "wasting and preoccupation caused by being shot by an elfin arrowhead."[55]

At the time that I was introduced to Elecampane, I was emerging from a period of my life in which I had tried to suppress my imagination and my spirituality to gain acceptance in relationships and in the culture around me. This meant denying fundamental aspects of both my childhood and adult experiences.

Elecampane can be a powerful ally in bringing gifts from the Otherworld—wisdom obtained through grief—back into this world, integrating spiritual awareness with physical reality, and bringing the spirit into the body. Breath is powerful for altering consciousness, and restoring the fluidity of breath can help someone to make the transition between different levels of reality more fluid. Just as Elecampane works at the physical level to resolve the associated respiratory disease, the plant can also help such a person bring the gifts gained from a lifetime of gazing into other realms more fully into this world, gaining confidence and stepping into power. Elecampane brings moisture up from damp soil to feed a bright yellow flower that grows high above the ground and invites us to choose to blossom in that same way.

For me, that choice involved coming more fully into my body and into this world without denying the reality of the music I heard from the other side of the veil. It meant allowing the Pagan concept of a living Earth that I professed to become real and embodied by listening to the forest and working with plants to bring healing to others and to myself. Elecampane gave me my breath. My breath gave me life.

Safety considerations: None.

Ecological considerations: Prolific in areas where it is wild or introduced and easily cultivated.

🌿 Ghost Pipe (*Monotropa uniflora*)

Strange and ethereal, Ghost Pipe emerges from beneath the forest floor in summer. Easily mistaken for a mushroom, Ghost Pipe is in fact a vascular plant with no chlorophyll whose white stalk blooms forth in a white blossom whose center becomes tinged with yellow pollen that attracts Bumblebees.

Ghost Pipe taps its roots into the place where the mycelium meets the rhizome, drawing off nutrients from mushroom and tree alike, and sends up a slender stalk that blossoms into a bell shape flower that first faces upward toward a sky whose sunlight it does not need and then nods down toward the ground that gives it life. Tapped into these nodes in the mycorrhizal network, Ghost Pipe is tapped into two very different systems for processing information—essentially two very different forms of consciousness. Mycelial consciousness is horizontal and diffuse—information is carried across vast networks of nerve-like filaments. Information moves rapidly and multi-directionally. But the web has no center where information can be concentrated and processed. In contrast, trees concentrate information over time in one place. The rings of their trunks holding the memory of rain and drought and fire. Plants and fungi exchange nutrients across their shared mycorrhizal networks. And in the process, they also exchange information in the form of chemical signals and in siphoning off nutrients from these mycorrhizal networks, Ghost Pipe is also tapping into the information they carry.

Ghost Pipe's white flower that blooms from beneath the earth to me brings a message that we can draw nourishment not only from the world of the living and the bright sun above, but also from the Otherworld. The mycorrhizal networks that sustain the plant include fungi (and depend on symbiotic bacteria) that metabolize the bodies of the dead, and hence their embodied memories. So too, we are nourished by the human and other-than-human ancestors who preceded us. Like the *Psilocybe* mushrooms, Ghost Pipe also teaches us that when our own forms dissolve the memories our bodies hold will become part of the memory of the Earth—a reality science is just catching up with as we learn to extract ancient genetic traces of skin and bone and saliva and sweat from soil. The soil is the fascia of the Earth, and the mycorrhizal network is akin to the collagen bundles that carry information in the form of light throughout the fascia.

Ghost Pipe's form resembles that of the spine and the brainstem. This signature points to an essential part of what the plant has to teach us: how to be at the nexus of worlds, listening to the voices above and the voices below and the voices around us without becoming overwhelmed. It teaches us to be aware of sensory and emotional inputs without being overwhelmed by them, how to engage them without identifying with them fully. This calls to mind the way in which the Irish language addresses emotion: we do not say *Is me brón* (I am sad), instead we say *Tá brón orm* (Sadness is upon me).

This is an essential skill in magical work. We have to be in touch with, aware of, the embodied sense of the presence of the beings we are working with, the currents of power around us, and the flow of sensation within us while still being able to maintain focused intention and conjure in our bodies the sense of motion toward the goal we and our magical partners are trying to achieve together. Ghost Pipe has been one of my most profound teachers in achieving this state.

Because Ghost Pipe is not a plant that can be planted or proliferated by humans, it is important to learn this from the plant without harvesting it. (I will not say that there is never a reason to work with this plant's physical medicine, but this is something I will only teach to people who have demonstrated an ability to listen deeply to plants and will only do myself when no other medicine and no other means of engaging it will do.) The best way to do this is to get down on the ground and be deeply present with the plant. Feel awareness go down from your root into the shared mycorrhizal network and focus on the presence of the plant before you. "Be still and know."

If you are called to bring the presence of the plant into your body, make a flower essence without harvesting the flower. On the night of the first crescent of the new moon, leave water in a stone vessel beside a grove of

Ghost Pipe. In the morning, come back for the water and combine it fifty-fifty with the alcohol that calls to you: brandy will preserve the essence in its purest form; a smoky, peaty whiskey can bring in some of the presence of ancient forests and fields. Work with the essence one drop at a time.

> **Safety considerations:** Theoretically there are a few constituents in this plant that can be dangerous: andromedotoxin and one or more cardiac glycosides. They exist in trace amounts and there are no accounts of poisoning with this plant (aside from one nineteenth-century account of a rash on the skin of a woman who had handled a specimen, but that rash was most likely actually caused by Poison Ivy.

> **Ecological considerations:** While locally abundant in some areas, this plant cannot be proliferated by humans, and I have seen overharvesting wipe entire populations out. The situations in which someone will actually need to harvest this plant are few and far between, and I will not address them in this book or in any broad public forum. When those situations do arise, taking only a few plants from a cluster and taking only the aerial parts, and working with the tincture at only very small doses is the most respectful way to work with Ghost Pipe's physical medicine.

❧ Goldenrod (*Solidago* spp.)

By the solar calendar, autumn is still a few weeks away. But here in Maine, summer is already fading—there is a soft golden light as afternoon turns to evening. Everywhere, Goldenrod blooms. It is abuzz with bees who will turn the nectar of the blossoms into sweet, amber honey.

Western Maine herbalist Gail Faith Edwards notes that Goldenrod is the last of the bright yellow flowers left blossoming in New England fields.[56] The medicine we make from it can bring sunlight into the darkness of winter, lifting the spirit. Restoring strength when energy is flagging is a keynote for Goldenrod's medicine. Matthew Wood writes:

All summer long, while other plants are flowering, Goldenrod is steadily raising its single stalk towards the sky. Finally, around the middle of August, the golden-yellow spires appear. Both a staff and a spire are included in the picture. It is like the tarot card showing a man walking along a road with a heavy burden on his back, a walking staff in his hand. His head is bent down, so that he does not see a church spire rising in the distance which shows that the distance is within his reach. The message of Goldenrod is to endure to reach the goal.[57]

Goldenrod is warming and sweetly aromatic. I harvest the flowers and leaves in fields where it is abundant, while focusing on the feeling of gratitude for the beauty and abundance of the wild world and praying to be strengthened in my resolve and ability to do the work I need to do make my contribution to the health of the land and her people. I tincture some in whiskey with a touch of honey to preserve its warmth and brightness and infuse some in oil.

A drop or two of the tincture will warm the weary spirit. Taking it in, I close my eyes and conjure the feeling of late summer sun warming my skin and imagine myself standing in a field of Goldenrod, inhaling its scent, as its body and my own release aromatic molecules called forth by heat and light.

Massaged into cold, stiff muscles, Goldenrod oil restores the flow of blood, awareness, and light. Light flows through the collagen fibers of our fascia when the muscles beneath it are relaxed, a network of photonic information transmission that parallels the electrical information transmission of our nerves. One of my favorite rituals is to lovingly anoint my body with Goldenrod oil and take a hot bath or shower. The heat drives the medicine deeper into my muscles. Then I invite my body to find the gentle, fluid movement that arises from being present in the moment.

Safety considerations: Be careful if you are allergic to other plants of the Asteraceae family, or if you are on medications for kidney disease or congestive heart failure. Otherwise, this is a very safe plant. Many people wrongly blame Goldenrod for their seasonal allergies because

it is blooming during a time when there are a lot of common allergens in the air, but its pollen is actually too heavy to be windborne.
Its gentle astringency does, however, make it an excellent medicine
for dealing with allergies involving red eyes and a drippy nose.

Ecological considerations: Abundant and prolific.

ஜ Hawthorn (*Crategus* spp.)

The mythic histories tell us that the arrival and decline of the Tuath Dé
was heralded by the blooming of the Hawthorn trees that grew upon the
hollow hills beneath which they disappeared as Celtic culture took hold.

On the morning of Bealtaine, the old celebration of Earth's ecstasy,
when the Hawthorn was in bloom—dew shimmering on its white
blossoms, suggesting the splendor of the fine raiments of the gentry—
people would tie ribbons to the tree with prayers for abundance and
hang cloths from its branches, which would be used later as bandages.
But the thorns of the Hawthorn suggested the wrath that would be
visited upon any who dared to damage it.

As late as the 1990s, folklorist Eddie Lenihan found many people
in the west of Ireland who shared stories of the woes that befell those
who damaged Hawthorns: one spoke of the tree beginning to bleed
when cut with a crosscut saw, another spoke of a man who, after cutting a Hawthorn, felt thorns in his bed every night for the rest of his
life. Those were among the milder consequences associated with such
desecration.[58] This recognition of Hawthorn's power arose from people
experiencing the world as alive and animated by quite different consciousnesses than their own.

But as fierce as Hawthorn can be in protecting the realm whose gates
it guards, when approached with respect, Hawthorn reveals a gentler side.
Victor Anderson said that the ways of the Tuath Dé and the Daoine Sidhe
were "kinder, and less civilized." Hawthorn helps prepare us to engage the
world in a way more similar to theirs. Hawthorn calms and strengthens
the heart and cools fires that burn too intensely in our blood vessels.

The heart moves out of balance, into excess, when our bodies and minds become overwhelmed with too much to process. We become agitated, unsettled, irritable, and reactive as our minds struggle to make meaning of what is happening around us. Our minds often end up spinning their wheels because they are not grounded in the present time and space—and because the amount and intensity of the information about potential threats they are dealing with and sensory stimuli that need to be deciphered exceeds their capacity.

That excited state is essentially the state we experience when we have too much caffeine—an alkaloid whose ubiquitous presence in our world has its roots in early capitalism and trade in beverages and foods made from stimulant plants Coffee (*Coffea arabica*), Tea (*Camellia sinensis*), and Cacao (*Theobroma cacao*) harvested from newly colonized lands. You can tell a lot about a culture by its drugs of choice. At moderate levels, caffeine makes people awake and focused. At higher doses, it makes many jittery and nervous. As the dose increases, caffeine increases the activity of norepinephrine, which makes us narrow our mental focus and increase our feelings of fear and aggression and inhibits serotonin, thus closing off more sensory information from the body and the world around it and decreasing nonlinear creativity. One French philosopher, living at the dawn of capitalism, who was known for drinking over five dozen cups of coffee in a day, infamously concluded that his thoughts—the belief structures and ideas of his talking self—were the primary confirmation of his existence. Descartes's ideas would define the emergence of a worldview that saw mind and body as separate and distinct entities and privileged rationality over emotion, intuition, and even empirical experience.

Like caffeine, fear can overwhelm us and trigger an increase of norepinephrine, narrowing the scope of and increasing the feverish speed of mental activity. Fear also curtails our capacity to make connections and our desire to seek connection, increasing alienation, which, in turn, increases fear and feeling overwhelmed.

Sometimes unrestrained panic, grief, and rage represent the same kind of revolution occurring within a person's being, her sensual and emotional wild self pushing against the rational structures imposed by the talking self and the demands enforced conformity imposes on our bodies. The upwelling of emotion breaks open a person's fixed sense of reality, creating the possibility of repressed emotions emerging and the transformation of a person's sense of being and meaning.

When it is not safe to simply release the barriers and allow "madness" to run its course, a safer and slower response is to work with gentle, subtly cooling, and grounding herbs to take the edge off the intensity of someone's experience. This allows them to move more smoothly through the experience of letting mental and emotional heat move through them and allowing them to return to grounded presence.

We are coming to understand the heart as a complex organ of perception that picks up on the subtle electromagnetic shifts that signal changes in our bodies and in the bodies of the living things around us. The heart relays these messages via the vagus nerve to the amygdala and to the right frontal cortex of the brain, where they are interpreted as emotion. In other words, the heart is just what our ancestors thought it was, an organ that shapes our felt sense of the world. In some ways, we can see the heart, the amygdala, and the right frontal cortex as forming an axis that is the physiological location of that aspect of our wild selves that seeks pleasure in connection.

Hawthorn's medicine is cool and dark, like the rich soil of an Apple orchard. It soothes the heart that is overheating from taking in too much from the outside world. What is too much? More than a person's amygdala and right frontal cortex can process. What situations will overwhelm a person vary widely, depending on how wide the sensory gates that allow information to pass from the heart to the brain are open, what associations he has with the sensations he is experiencing, and how much unprocessed emotion is held inside his body.

I love to tincture the leaf, flower, and berry together in a good Irish whiskey with a touch of honey and include a single thorn. I will mix a little of the tincture with heavy cream when making offerings to the tree, my Irish ancestors, or the Daoine Sidhe.

I learned from Matthew Wood that Hawthorn is specific for reducing "heat and irritation in the capillaries."[59] This explains the medicine's well-known ability to mitigate cardiovascular disease and also relates to its use in managing inflammation in the respiratory and digestive tracts, and its possible relevance in helping to manage the body's response to COVID-19 infection, as well as managing our responses to a world full of things that inflame our minds, our senses, and our tissues.

Hawthorn wasn't used for cardiovascular issues in the West until the early twentieth century, but it was widely used in medieval Europe to aid in the digestion of meat. Similarly, Hawthorn is used in Chinese medicine to treat indigestion.

In the 1990s, Dr. Deborah Frances pioneered the use of Hawthorn in the treatment of acute asthma attacks marked by "constriction and tightness in the chest."[60] I've found it especially useful for asthma attacks brought on by emotional triggers and often preceded by heat in the cheeks and earlobes.

I am wary of making leaps from the conclusions of in vitro and animal studies of plant constituents to practical use of an herb with people, but when they line up with traditional knowledge of a plant and my own empirical experience, the three sets of evidence support and confirm each other. So it is with the research around Hawthorn and inflammation. I will just go into the basics here.

Hawthorn reduces inflammation in the epithelial cells of the lining of the respiratory tract and the walls of the blood vessels by preventing proinflammatory cytokines from recruiting white blood cells to the area. One Hawthorn constituent, vitexin, has been shown to act in a similar way to mediate inflammation in the respiratory tract.

Some polyphenols from Hawthorn also appear to inhibit ACE (angiotensin-converting enzyme), thereby weakening the action of angiotensin, a hormone that signals the body to constrict the blood vessels. Constricting blood vessels raises blood pressure and can also increase local inflammation by impeding healthy circulation. ACE converts raw angiotensin 1 into the active form of angiotensin, angiotensin 2.

ACE has a counterpart, ACE2, which deactivates angiotensin 2, relaxing and opening the blood vessels.

This is particularly relevant in dealing with COVID-19, a virus whose actions, I think, in many ways mirror and are exacerbated by our cultural tendency toward inflammatory responses to the world, both literal and figurative (which are ultimately one and the same—physiological inflammation brings inflammatory emotional responses, which create more stress, which creates more physiological inflammation). COVID-19 attaches itself to ACE2 receptors, initially in the lung, which interferes with the action of ACE2, thus increasing the action of angiotensin 2, causing blood vessels to constrict, spiking blood pressure, and causing tissue damage up to and including respiratory failure, scarring of the lung tissue, myocarditis, and kidney failure. Researchers are exploring whether flooding the body with ACE2 might be an effective way of treating COVID-19.

I don't know of any herbs that boost ACE2 levels, but in Hawthorn (and in Reishi), we have herbs that could theoretically help tilt the balance slightly in the right direction by inhibiting ACE and thus reducing levels of angiotensin 2 and somewhat reducing the need for ACE2. We also have other herbs that we know are vasodilators—like Black Cohosh, Yarrow, and Lobelia—that combine beautifully with Hawthorn. Vasodilating herbs have the added benefit of being diaphoretics, herbs that allow the body to disperse heat.

What happens with our breath effects our heart rate. What happens with the rhythm of the physical heart effects the emotional heart. This is not a metaphor. I work with Hawthorn when the outside world is overwhelming. Emotion and sensation build to a point when a person's internal processing becomes less and less coherent, and the body's inflammatory responses begin to kick in. Very often the person's ears will become hot and will even visibly redden just before the building heat triggers an undirected explosive expression—a combined implosion and explosion, which could express itself as an inflammatory asthma attack or as a cessation of verbal communication but with the body moving involuntarily with the force of the sensation moving through it (which should never be forcibly stopped).

Matthew Wood notes that Hawthorn is especially well suited for mental and emotional agitation in Autistic and other neurodivergent people who, in Celtic cultures, would have been identified as Faerie changelings, children from another world. He also notes that Hawthorn is heavily associated with the Faerie realm in folklore. Because Hawthorn guards the gate between this world and the Faerie world and so is well suited to those whose neurobiology naturally resists the tight regulation of consciousness imposed by our culture. Hawthorn cools the heart and the blood to make us more receptive and less reactive to the world.

> **Safety considerations:** Use caution if you have low blood pressure or are taking medications to lower your blood pressure. Do not harm a Hawthorn.
>
> **Ecological considerations:** Most species are fairly abundant in the areas where they are native or introduced, though some native species on the North American Pacific coast are being squeezed out by introduced species. Fairly easily cultivated.

꧁ Lady's Slipper (*Cypripedium acaule*)

Walking in the forest in late May, the sight of the first Lady Slipper in bloom always brings me to my knees. The gasp it brings is in part the awe I feel in the presence of the sacred—but something else as well: an ecstasy tinged with astonishment felt not just by the spirit but by the body as a whole, most markedly at the heart, the diaphragm, and the root of myself. A bliss of the embodied spirit taking pure delight in the sensual pleasure of the gorgeousness of the flower.

This is the response that the flower evolved to elicit. The beauty of the flower exists for the purpose of seduction—drawing in bees whose wings and bodies are dusted with the pollen of another Lady's Slipper, which will fertilize the ovum that will become the seed in autumn. Our biology is not that different from that of the bees. We too are seduced by pink blossoms in the forest and fall in wild, unbridled love with the flowers and the forest that gives them life.

Kate Gilday writes that Pink Lady's Slipper flower essence aids with "releasing shame" and "understanding and delight in one's sexuality, opening one to deeper levels of intimacy."[61] This speaks of a return to innocence in its deepest sense—the state of being without guilt, shame, or fear, free to follow the authentic response we feel to the world from the heart and from the root. In this culture, we tend to think of innocence as something that can never be regained once it is lost. But true innocence is always available to us through coming back to our true selves and coming back into relation with our wild kindred. Victor Anderson connected this concept with the word *sankofa* from the cultures of Central Africa, from which his most important teacher descended. Anderson said that Sankofa, a concept symbolized by a black heart ("the Black Heart of Innocence" he called it) or a bird looking backward and holding an egg in a posture that puts the bird's body into the shape of a heart, means that "it is not wrong to go back for that which you have forgotten."[62] We fail to go back for that which we have forgotten at our own peril. Lady's Slipper helps us remember how to do this, how to respond to the world with joy and wonder.

Stephen Harrod Buhner describes the medicine of Lady's Slipper as being like two loving hands cradling the heart. I learned from him that in the wake of the Civil War, the shattered hearts of soldiers cried out for the Lady's Slipper's medicine, and she was gathered almost to the point of extinction.

Plant medicines produce a direct and immediate impact in the body to alleviate suffering. At the same time they work to help the body remember the way back to health. This deep and often subtle healing happens best when space is opened for the plant to work deeply inside someone over time, penetrating further into the consciousness and the heart field. These forms of healing are, of course, inextricably linked. But in a culture that has forgotten that the plants are our ancestors and teachers, the living medicine of the plants we use is often forgotten and ignored. Too often, plant medicines are applied in a mechanistic way to create a specific result in the body. The medicine is still the medicine, but when we don't give it space and time to do its work and we don't engage the plant, much is lost.

I imagine the shape of the Lady's Slipper's blossom—a heart open in the center shielded by winglike petals—and I imagine the way she could teach a heart forced shut by the brutality of war to begin to allow healing in again. And knowing many veterans who left pieces of themselves on distant battlefields, I also know something of the incredible patience and strength that opening takes.

Did the doctors treating "soldier's heart" in the wake of the Civil War bring their patients to the woods to be with the plants that would become their medicine? More likely, the tinctured or powdered root was administered to a patient who was taught little about its source. In the parlance of the day the plant was known as American Valerian, used primarily as a sedative. Plants are generous, using their bodies to create the medicines that will restore the imbalances in the ecosystem they perceive through the chemical and electromagnetic information they take in from the world around them—including the imbalances in the bodies of the humans who share their habitat. But the imbalances created in our culture are too big for the plants to correct through chemistry alone.

There weren't enough Lady's Slippers in all of North America to heal all the pain and terror and loss the people here experienced as a result of the Civil War. And at the same time a single Lady's Slipper could have taught the culture all it needed to know about how to reshape itself in ways that would give hearts the space they needed to heal and open again like pink orchids in the understory of a shady forest.

It still can. Lady's Slipper is a plant whose medicine is best experienced through direct presence and through the somatic memory of the late spring day when you first come upon her in the forest. If you must call upon her in another way and another time, work with a flower essence made without harvesting the flower. Place a bowl of water beneath the blossom in the early morning and come back to gather the water just before dusk. Combine with an equal part of brandy to preserve it.

> **Safety considerations:** Harvesting a plant so rare places one in spiritual danger.
>
> **Ecological considerations:** This is a rare flower that depends on very particular mycorrhizal relationships to thrive that are next to impossible to replicate outside its natural environment. I am only aware of a very small number of instances in which it has been successfully cultivated. The only way to ethically harvest this flower and its root, which is the source of its physiological medicine, is to do so from places that are about to be bulldozed or clear-cut.

🌿 Lobelia (*Lobelia inflata*)

Lobelia is the quintessential herb for relaxing tension. Matthew Wood recently described it to me as the herb that awakens the autonomic nervous system and hence the Animal Self. I think of it is as the key that unlocks the cage that tension has created to contain the Animal Self. This means, of course, you have to be somewhat careful with it because sometimes a caged animal runs for the forest when set free, but sometimes that caged animal responds with fear and rage pent up during the time of its imprisonment. Lobelia first entered the pharmacopeia of the English-speaking world through the work of the cantankerous New Hampshire farmer and herbalist Samuel Thomson in the early years of the current republic. Thomson used it to clear the way for the fire of the body to burn away illness.

Most people, on taking Lobelia, feel an irritation in the back of their throat. The herb stimulates the acrid taste receptors, resetting the signal the vagus nerve carries through the body and restoring channels of communication among the major centers of our nervous system (the brain, the heart, the gut, and the genitals), reaffirming safety, inviting us to enter an open and relaxed state. This is followed by the action of the alkaloid lobeline on receptors. It further encourages the release of tension without sedating awareness, an action similar to that of nicotine in the body. This alkaloid also works synergistically with acetylcholine to help consolidate learning and memory. Nicotine does the same thing, but with nicotine, there is damage to the receptor sites for acetylcholine, which can lead, over time, to cognitive decline. With Lobelia there is no such damage. Lobeline also helps the body slow the conversion of dopamine—which is involved in the creation of motivation, reward, and meaning—to norepinephrine, which narrows the focus and creates anxiety when its levels are too high. For this reason, I use the herb not only with anxious people but also with people whose flat depression follows a period of intense stress, which led to a depletion of dopamine. In these instances, I like to combine it with high doses of the dopaminergic herb Brahmi (*Bacopa monnieri*) and Damiana (*Turnera diffusa*), which inhibits MAO-B, the sister enzyme of MAO-A. MAO-A breaks down all of our major neurotransmitters, but MAO-B breaks down only dopamine, so inhibiting MAO-B will tilt the balance in favor of dopamine. (More on this above, under the Damiana section.)

Take a moment to think about the places where you see people smoking Tobacco most frequently: outside veterans' halls, twelve-step meetings, and emergency rooms. In war zones and prisons. In bus stations and back alleys. People smoke Tobacco in these situations because they need to release tension without losing their focus on their surroundings. Most people in these same situations will benefit from Lobelia.

The second thing most people experience when they take Lobelia is an expansion of the airways, a relaxation and opening of the chest, and a softening of the diaphragm. This allows the breath and the heart rate to normalize, helping someone become more present in their body. The sense of opening it brings to the chest is similar to that brought by stimulating the Pericardium 6 (PC 6) acupuncture point or *nei guan* (inner gate), which lies three finger-widths down from the scaphoid between the tendons of the wrist. The pericardium, in Chinese medicine, is the heart protector, and both drop doses of Lobelia and stimulation of PC 6 help to reopen someone's awareness to what is present here and now. I've had particularly good results applying a drop of Lobelia directly to that acupuncture point. The physical pericardium, which holds and supports the physical heart, rests only when the heart is supported by the diaphragm during the brief pause we take between inhalation and exhalation. I experience particularly strong opening up of the breath and of awareness when, while applying Lobelia to PC 6, I also lengthen the pause between inhalation and exhalation. I suspect the combination helps to restore heart rate variability.

Lobelia is also an herb I use in emergency situations to open the airways. The flowers of the species were considered "official" in the pharmacopeia until it was deemed "too capricious" and removed from use in conventional medicine. *Lobelia inflata* has flowers whose form resembles the air sacs in the lung. Some herbalists favor the *Ephedra* genus, an emergency bronchodilator, but *Ephedra* and its eponymous alkaloid, ephedrine, open the airways by stimulating the sympathetic nervous system response, inducing anxiety.

Lobelia is often one of the first herbs that I will give someone because it brings them into a clear, grounded presence, which opens the way for other medicines to move through the body. Most formulae I make have at least a little bit of Lobelia for that purpose.

I have also worked with Lobelia ritually in situations where constrictions and restrictions block the path forward. My simplest way of working with any plant magically is to take a drop of a tincture, a sip of tea, or a puff of smoke into my body and ask the plant spirit to instruct me how to deal with the situation at hand.

> **Safety considerations:** Too large a dose will make you vomit, which makes it hard for this herb to cause physical poisoning. It is a very safe medicine.
> **Ecological considerations:** Prolific in the wild and easily cultivated.

🌿 Motherwort (*Leonurus cardiaca*)

In the midst of a winter rainstorm, at a time when my life was in turmoil, a woman I was just beginning to know—whom I now count as a dear *cara anam,* a friend of my soul—welcomed me in from the road with a cup of Motherwort tea. After drinking the tea, we lay beside the woodstove, speaking of selkies—the shape-shifting seal people of Irish and Scottish (and Maine and Nova Scotia) legend—and singing sweet, haunting old ballads, while her young son slept nearby. I will always remember the gentle warmth of that night and the way I was able to put aside all my worries and allow myself to accept shelter and care. Every time I taste Motherwort, I feel like I am being tenderly held and nourished. It soothes my spirit deeply.

Like Damiana, Motherwort works with oxytocin to bring us into a place where we can receive affection and care and feel connection. But while Damiana stimulates the circulation, arousing us to movement, Motherwort soothes a heart that is beating too hard and too fast, allowing us to relax into presence and, sometimes, into sleep. Yet Motherwort will also just as easily nourish and revive a weary heart.

Motherwort reminds us that mother is a verb that means to give life and to love and care for that life unconditionally. It is the hand of the God Self reaching down to replenish and settle the waters of the Cauldron of Motion.

As I mentioned earlier, regarding the Cauldron of Motion, Motherwort is especially indicated where sudden surges of emotion bring heat, blood, and redness rising to the head and seek release in hot tears. I have sometimes even been able to visually observe the process of that blood flushing the neck and the face and then, with a few drops of Motherwort, draining back down.

This downward direction of the blood flow is a property of many of the bitter mints that act on the nervous system—Motherwort, Lemon Balm, Skullcap, Wood Betony—though each does so in subtly different ways. Lemon Balm calms flashes of anger and also helps when too much sun makes someone irritable. Skullcap brings blood flow from an overactive brain down to the abdomen. And Wood Betony anchors all three selves firmly in the solar plexus to protect us from outside influences and ground us in the here and now.

Safety considerations: None.

Ecological considerations: Prolific in areas where it is wild or
introduced and easily cultivated.

🌿 Mullein (*Verbascum thapsus*)

Mullein stands tall and erect, giving rise to a torch of brilliant yellow
flowers that blaze brightly in the misty Maine morning even after everything else in the field has died back. Gazing at it, I find my spine aligning with its stalk, my breath deepening, my mind clearing. I become my
own axis mundi, my own world tree, rooted in the earth, growing upward
toward the sky, allowing air and water to move through me more freely.

For me, much of Mullein's medicine and magic are about alignment.
Matthew Wood is largely responsible for resurrecting the use of Mullein as
an herb for acute musculoskeletal injury and especially for helping bones
heal in their proper alignment. Generally, I use the leaf for this purpose,
but I learned from jim mcdonald that Mullein root is specific for issues of
the lower spine—the root of the first year's growth of this biennial plant,
which would give rise to the upright stalks of the next season were it left
in the ground to grow. The great seventeenth-century herbalist Nicholas
Culpepper used Mullein seed for a similar purpose: "The seed bruised and
boiled in wine, and laid on any member that has been out of joint, and
newly set again, takes away all swelling and pain thereof."[63] Wood specu-
lates that Mullein is acting to restore the proper flow of synovial fluid to
the connective tissues, allowing them to better support proper regrowth
of the bone, especially if administered in conjunction with Solomon's Seal.
Mullein's role as a lymph mover may also be at work here, allowing the
metabolic wastes produced in the process of tissue repair to move out of
the tissues and reducing swelling that might impinge on proper alignment.

There is also an element of Mullein's medicine of alignment that
defies a rationalist materialist explanation. Margi Flint taught me that
a Mullein stalk hung over or placed under the bed will improve spinal
alignment. I was skeptical until I noticed that every time I sat under the

Mullein stalk she had hanging from her rafters I sat up straighter! And sitting up straighter, I felt more clearheaded.

I suspect some of Mullein leaf's ability to help heal old coughs, in addition to involving the herb's ability to help restore the proper viscosity to the respiratory mucosa through its joint action on the kidneys and the lungs, probably has to do with this capacity to restore proper pliability to connective tissues as well. The chest needs to be able to expand and contract fully for healthy breath. Spinal alignment and proper posture are also essential for deep breathing as well.

Mullein leaf, of course, also helps the lungs directly. Always among the first plants to grow up in the wake of a wildfire, I find that smoking Mullein leaves or drinking the finely strained infusion of the leaves can be incredibly helpful in healing lungs damaged by smoke inhalation—whether from woodstoves or wildfires or Tobacco smoking, the medicine of a burned over place aiding burned over tissues.

Mullein root is a powerful astringent, which Culpepper used in treating dysentery and urinary tract obstructions: "The decoction of the root in red wine or in water, (if there be an ague) wherein red hot steel hath been often quenched, doth stay the bloody-flux. The same also opens obstructions of the bladder and reins[kidneys]."[64] More recently, several herbalists have used either the tincture or the decoction of Mullein root to tonify the bladder sphincter in cases of urinary incontinence. When using it for this purpose, I often also give Nettle seed (*Urtica dioscia*) to strengthen the kidneys and Schisandra (*Schisandra chinensis*) as an astringent with a strong kidney affinity. I have combined it with my three main urinary tract antispasmodics—Kava, Cannabis, and Wild Yam—in cases where prolonged and frequent ketamine use has resulted in partial paralysis of the bladder sphincter.

Mullein emerges as a plant that helps to bring focused presence when we look at these aspects of the medicine together: Mullein root astringes us at the root, stopping the leaking of energy; Mullein root and leaf improve spinal alignment; and Mullein leaf and flower ease respiration—along with Mullein's gentle capacity to soothe an irritated nervous system and allay pain. This also relates to Mullein as a traditional herb of protection: being grounded and present and aligned in the fullness of who we are is the best protection against curses consciously and unconsciously sent our way. Having established that prayer, focused goodwill, has the power to heal, we have to acknowledge the corollary—that strong ill will can knock us off balance. Being centered is the best way to avoid being swayed by such ill winds.

Thomas Oswald Cockayne's nineteenth-century translation of an Anglo-Saxon Materia Medica tells us:

> It is said that Mercurius should give this wort to Ulixes, the chieftain, when he came to Circe, and he after that dreaded none of her works. . . . If one beareth with him one twig of this wort, he will not be terrified with any awe, nor will a wild beast hurt him, or any evil coming near.[65]

Irish folklorist Niall Mac Coitir notes: "The name 'hag's taper' [common in Ulster] derives from the belief that mullein was a favorite plant for witches to use for wicks in their lanterns and candles when casting spells."[66] This also suggests to me a focusing of the will—gathering the energy and moving it upward to the point of focus, the fire in the head, just as the wick draws on the oil of the lamp to feed the flame. We can think of the spine as the wick of the fire of consciousness.

Mullein is the plant of healthy alignment. Physical alignment opens the way for spiritual alignment. As my spine straightens in alignment with the Mullein growing in the field, my heart speaks the words of Victor Anderson's prayer: "May all three souls be straight within me." I breathe deeply, root down, stand tall, and allow life to flow through me in the way that is right and true. Then, like Mullein flowers in late summer, I shine brightly in the world.

Safety considerations: The fine hairs of the leaf can be irritating.
Ecological considerations: Prolific, common, and resilient.

❧ Nettles (*Urtica dioica*)

Nettles are at once nourishing and purifying. It's the perfect herb for helping the body navigate the transition from winter to spring, when they are one of the first wild greens present in abundance. I give them not as a drop dose tincture but as a tea or a food—and sometimes use them to sting myself, but we will get to that in a bit.

Nettle leaf soup, made with cream and butter and sometimes seaweed, has nourished people in Ireland for thousands of years. Nettles are astoundingly nutritious. They contain more than three times as much protein and more than seventy-five times as much iron as Wheat or Barley and are also rich in calcium, magnesium, potassium, and vitamin C. The milk fat in the cream and butter in the soup aids in the absorption of many of those nutrients. Seaweed would add even more minerals.

Legend tells us that Saint Colm Cille, the "Dove of the Church," exiled from Ireland to the island of Iona, was out walking one fine spring day and saw an old woman gathering Nettles. He asked her why she was doing this, and she told him that she mostly survived on Nettle soup. He then vowed to eat nothing but Nettle soup himself. A concerned monk convinced Colm Cille to allow him to prepare the soup, though, and secretly added broth to it each day.

If I were to put a client on a mono-diet, bone broth with Nettles would absolutely be my first choice. So too for my ancestors. Winter in the Irish countryside was traditionally a time of long nights spent around peat fires, taking shelter from the wind and the rain. When spring came, Nettle soup helped get the blood moving again. Irish folklorist Niall Mac Coitir writes: "Nettle was considered to be good for purifying the blood, and it was widely believed in Ireland that taking three meals of Nettles in May guarded against illness for the next year."[67]

We now know, of course, that Nettles help the liver build blood proteins while helping the kidneys remove excess proteins (including metabolic wastes and allergens) from the blood—making them both a blood builder and a blood cleanser in a much more literal way than we usually mean when we use such terms. It is also an amazing hemostatic herb, helping to staunch blood loss. Dr. Kenneth Proefrock notes that thinking and worrying are metabolic activities that produce a significant amount of proteinaceous waste. Mac Coitir adds: "In west Galway, the man of the house would go out on May Eve and gather a handful of nettles. The nettles were pressed, and everyone in the house would drink a mouthful of the juice to 'keep a good fire in them' the rest of the year."[68] That particular turn of phrase, "keep a good fire in them," suggests Nettles role in bringing motion back to the middle cauldron. It also reflects an understanding of the way that Nettles both help to fuel our metabolic fires and clear their "ash" in order to keep them burning cleanly.

Nettles certainly get the blood flowing when they sting! There is a popular saying in Gaeilge—*Neantóg a dhóigh mé agus cupóg a leigheas mé*: "Nettle burned me, and Dock cured me." Nettles and Dock often grow side by side, and a poultice of Dock leaves helps bring down the heat and intensity of a Nettle sting. (Plantain, *Plantago major*, leaves make an even more effective poultice for Nettle stings, and there is some speculation that the saying may have initially referred not to Dock but to Plantain, Slánlus in Irish.) But not everyone wants to avoid Nettle stings! Because they do get the blood flowing, Nettle stings are a tried-and-true remedy for arthritis and gout. I have also found them a great remedy for the lethargy and depression that linger longer into springtime from winter than feels right. It is a powerful shock of electricity that can waken a nervous system or shock it into the present moment. A few drops of Lobelia will make the body even more receptive, and a few drops of Prickly Ash can bring a complementary stimulation and help the current move more efficiently through the body.

Mac Coitir reports another Irish Nettle tradition:

In southern parts of County Cork, May Eve was known as "Nettlemas Night," when boys would parade the streets with large bunches of Nettles, stinging their playmates and occasionally unfortunate passersby who got too close. Girls would join in too, stinging their lovers or boys for whom they held affection.[69]

Nettle stings bring an intense sensation and a rush of energy. If the Nettle leaves are a fitting medicine for the spring equinox, the Nettle sting certainly has a fitting place in youthful rites at Lá Bealtaine, with all their wild innocence.

Not all of Nettle's associations in Ireland are quite so joyful. During the An Gorta Mór, the Great Hunger, in the 1840s, a million Irish died of starvation and disease and a million more fled for England, Canada, or the United States or were shipped as prisoners to Australia—all while the occupying British continued to export thousands of shiploads of food grown on Irish soil to London, Liverpool, and Glasgow. Even today, the landscape in the west of Ireland is marked by the foundations of tumbledown cottages— remnants of that period—now grown over with Nettles. So common is the sight, that examples of the use of the word *neantóga* include *tá neantóga san áit a raibh an teach tráth* and *tá neantóga mar a raibh an teach tráth*—two ways of saying "there are Nettles where the house once was."

But Nettles also represent resilience. Few people know that the Great Hunger was in part a long-term consequence of the British campaign of deforestation that all but eradicated Ireland's great Oak and Hazel forests, depriving people of the Deer and Boar they once hunted and the Hazelnuts they once gathered. This deforestation also silted the streams where Salmon once swam and let the wind and rain sweep the soil into the sea. This soil depletion made Ireland's small farms especially susceptible to disasters like the blight that struck the potatoes in the 1840s. Nettles are famous for their ability to grow in and restore fertility to poor soils. Along with seaweed, they are one of the wild foods that kept many alive through the Great Hunger.

Peadar Kearney, an Irish songwriter born a generation later, saw the spirit of Ireland as an old woman gathering Nettles while remembering the glories and mourning the loss of Irish men who had died in the country's many uprisings.[70]

> *'Twas down by the glenside,*
> *I met an old woman,*

A-plucking young nettles,
Nor thought I was coming
I listened awhile
To the song she was humming,
"Glory O, glory O,
To the Bold Fenian men!"
'Tis fifty long years
since I saw the moon beaming
And strong manly forms,
Their eyes with hope gleaming
I see them again
Sure, through all my days dreaming,
"Glory O, glory O,
To the Bold Fenian men!"

The Fenians were rebels who took their name from the Fianna, bands of warriors who lived in the forest, serving no one chieftain or province, but instead defending the land and the people. They were also trained as ecstatic poets, and the visions they experienced in the forest would guide their actions in protecting the vulnerable. The first Fianna were trained by Fionn mac Cumhail, a warrior who had gained wisdom in his youth by accidentally eating the first bit of oil that splattered from the body of the Salmon from the Otherworld Well that his Druid teacher had caught and asked him to prepare.

In Kearney's time, another generation of Fenians rose up and won independence for all but Northern Ireland in Na Cogadh na Saoirse (the War of Freedom). He fought among them and wrote the national anthem for the Irish Republic. The republic the former Fenian soldiers formed emerged on an island ecologically devastated by centuries of intensive occupation and exploitation. Perhaps if left to do their work, the Nettles will, in time, regenerate the land that so many generations fought to see free.

Safety considerations: Nettle stings can be uncomfortable but are generally salutary.

Ecological considerations: Abundant.

❧ Oak (*Quercus spp.*)

An old Oak grows outside the house where I grew up. As a child, I saw the black scar left by a fallen bough as a portal to the Otherworld. I came to this intuitively, and only as an adult did I learn that this aligned with very old lore about the Oak. Erynn Rowan Laurie writes:

> For me, as for many others, Oak also has links to gateways and thresholds—the liminal places where you are neither inside nor out, not in one place or another, but somewhere in between. It is in those edge-places where profound meetings with deity can occur. It's a place where wisdom, insight, and the understanding to provide a true judgment can be found.[71]

Niall Mac Coitir writes about the young lovers, Diarmaid and Grainne, fleeing the wrath of the elderly King Fionn to whom Grainne had been promised:

> A poem in the *Metrical Dindshenchas* about the Slige Dála talks about the ancient lore of Samhain being learned in oakwood's spirits and fairy folk. In "The Pursuit of Diarmaid and Gráinne," the pair stop at a place called Doire Dá Bhaoth (Oakwood of the Two Fools) and Diarmaid cuts seven doors of wood from the grove to protect them. These may have had magical significance as the Fianna are unable to pass through them and are forced to wait for Diarmaid to come out. There is also a play on words here between doire (oak grove) and doirse (doors).[72]

The Oak is associated with the letter *dair* in the old Irish Ogham alphabet, which corresponds to the letter *D*. Dair remains the name of the Oak in the modern Irish language, cognate with the Welsh *dár* and *derwen,* which refers specifically to the White Oak, both the species of that name and the twin of the Oak that grows in Annwn, the Welsh Otherworld. It is connected in Irish with the word *draoi,* which refers to one who works magic, and with its Welsh cognate *derwydd,* literally "Oak-seer," which is both the root of the modern word *druid* and the Welsh word for a prophet-poet, kin to the Irish *fili.* In the Arthurian tales, the Oak is the tree in which Myrddin (Merlin) sleeps waiting for the time when his magic will be called for again. That the Oak is also associated with sacral kingship in Irish, Scottish, and Welsh cultures points to the possibility that the kingly Arddur or Arthur and the sorcerous Myrddin were perhaps once two aspects or roles of one being, split in two by the coming of Christianity, and then departing the world to return in its time of great need. If ever there were a time of such need it is now, and I look to the Oak as a teacher of forgotten ways of being. As did Gwydion Pendderwen, great bard of the Feri tradition, who Victor Anderson adopted as his spiritual son. His chosen surname, Pendderwen, means "Master of the White Oak." He died in 1982, and I often feel his spirit close at Samhain.

The Oak is indeed a bridger of worlds. A mighty late succession tree in hardwood forests throughout North America, Asia, and Europe, the Oak roots deeply, drawing up ancient waters from deep in the earth, and sends branches up high, its crowns becoming the canopy of the forest, drawing down sunlight and rain from above. In Celtic, Germanic, and Scandinavian cultures, it is said to be "the lightning tree," conducting the sudden surges of power between worlds. The Oak can survive a lightning strike, its trunk becoming forked where it was struck. In Norse traditions, this is connected with the blow of Thor's hammer; in Irish tradition, it is associated with the blow of the Dagda's axe. The Dagda, one of the leaders of the Tuath Dé, made both his great weapon, a mighty club, and his harp, which could call people to laugh or to mourn or to sleep, from Oak wood.

The words for *door* and *Oak* have been near homophones in some Proto-Indo-European languages for as far back as we know. Interestingly, the association with the letter *D* and the passage between realms exists in the unrelated Semitic languages as well, with *daleth,* the fourth letter of the Hebrew alphabet, representing the gateway between form and matter in the kabbalah. Victor Anderson told Cornelia Benavidez about this connection and that it had to do with the primal connection between sound and shape:

> Everything has a voice, a tone, a symbol which is a part of its own shape. So, it is true that the Druids were the flower of the same kind of tradition which I have. They are the flower of that as it existed in the forests of ancient Europe and also in other places. And the name Druid means like I say the oak tree, the tree of life, the tree of knowledge and so forth. And there's something that must be understood by everyone now, although it used to be kept rather secret: "Druid" is spelled "D-R-U-I-D." That D is a door from the Hebrew DALETH which means door, path and to flow. There's the second D. We flow from one place to another; we do this all the time. We are born, we are reborn, we progress, and so that's what the word really means. And there are different variations. In ancient India, we had the word "druma" and which means something like, in fact it does mean "Tree."[73]

Old Irish lore supports this idea, with the *Metrical Dindshenchas,* a collection of Old Irish poems containing the lore of place names, telling us that sound and matter are the mother and father of Ogham, brought together by the third force of the twig held in the hand of the god Ogma. Physics tells us that states of matter are related to the rate of vibration of that matter. Wood makes sound as it changes temperature or moves with the wind. The letter *D* is a solid sound that creates a container for the open sounds of the vowels that precede or follow it. As such it suits the solidity of Oak—which has long been a favored wood for the making of doors because that solidity provides the ability to keep out what needs to be kept out and keep in what needs to be kept in until Will directs us to unbar the door and let it move on its hinges. Interestingly, this also corresponds to the physiological medicine of Oak, with its tannins increasing the integrity of epithelial tissue, the boundary and gate of our organs and our bodies themselves.

The solidity of the Oak is deeply nurturing and protective. Lean back against the body of an Oak, and you will feel your full weight supported. Supported and protected, you can ground in the earth, sending tendrils of your own consciousness down from your root to braid with the roots and rhizomes of the Oak. Follow those rhizomes, and you can tap into the mycorrhizal network, the mind of the forest. The wood of the Oak is a repository of the memory of that mind, carrying memories of sunlight and rain and snow over centuries or even millennia. To be an Oak-seer is to take a long view of the arc of history, rooted in the history of the land itself.

Like the Dagda whose cauldron feeds all who come to his feast, the Oak is also a generous provider. Acorns feed creatures great and small from the tiniest Mouse to the great Bear. Place Acorns on your altar to bring a reminder of that generosity—and then return them, blessed by your prayers, to the place you found them, that they might feed your wild kin in the dark winter to come.

Safety considerations: None.

Ecological considerations: Abundant where it has not been felled. The clearing of Ireland's Oak forests was a conscious act of cultural genocide and ecocide during the reign of Elizabeth I of England.

🌿 Pine (*Pinus* spp.)

Walking in the Maine woods in winter, the same snow that muffles the sound of distant traffic amplifies the song of the wind blowing through the Pines. The cold, crisp air is filled with their scent.

The Scots traditionally called the Pine *an clársach nan craobh*— the harp of the trees.[74] Cornelia Benavidez says that her mother and grandmother taught her that in Germany the sound of the wind in the

Pines and the scent of the tree were said to soothe a troubled mind. From what little I understand of their traditions, the Wabanaki peoples, whose homeland I inhabit, have similar teachings about the medicine of the Pine tree's presence.

In the Ogham, the Pine and the Fir, which are interchangeably called *ochtacht* in Old Irish, are associated with the letter *ailm*. Laurie writes:

> Ailm is the "ah!" cry of birth and death. (McManus . . . says that the word Ailm's meaning is uncertain, though all the word ogams point to a meaning of the "ah" sound itself, hence my use of "Cry"; for its definition.) It is a kind of initiation, where birth and death are one, a passage from one state to another. Its keyword is inception, and it indicates beginnings. Where Beith indicates primacy and the importance of what comes first, Ailm is beginning in its purest form. It is origin and creation.[75]

It is also inspiration, the literal and figurative breathing in of spirit that feeds the fires of creation within us. Breath is a thread that connects us with the life of the world. We breathe together with the forest, our exhalations becoming the inhalations of the trees, their exhalations becoming our inhalations. What we breathe out carries something of our inner world into the Great World beyond, what we breathe in carries something of the Great World into our inner world. Robin Artisson speaks of the breath soul we breathe in at birth:

> The breath soul is created by the body's relationship to the air that surrounds the world: the wind of this world or the greater envelope of air that encases the earth. When a newborn child breathes air in for the first time, a tiny portion of the "wind of the world" is captured and carries life-vitality into the baby's body. This vitalizing force personalizes in intimate respiratory contact with the child, and very rapidly, the breath soul (which constantly moves in and out of a breathing being's body) becomes a familiar and necessary presence in the body-soul complex, supplying vitality and animating life-donation

to the entire living system of a person. If the breath soul is lost or prevented from entering and leaving the body, the being will rapidly die. It can be lost briefly, in moments of breathlessness or "having the wind knocked out of a person"—resulting in a swift and painful struggle to think straight or maintain consciousness.[76]

This corresponds with the talking self or Human Self. Victor Anderson told Cornelia Benavidez that in the Hawai'ian tradition, this is called "the Uhane, the shining soul, (also spirit soul), which is the same thing as the Jewish 'Ruah' (life spirit)."[77] *Ruah* is a Hebrew word meaning "breath" or "spirit." Genesis 1:2 refers to the Ruach Elohim—the breath of the divine (referred to in this case by a linguistically plural name), which is a wind that moves over the water, bringing life.

In the Orkneys, Pine or Fir candles are used in a *saining* or ritual purification of a newborn: the resinous, flaming candle is whirled around the bed three times. This is similar to the use of Myrrh to bless a newborn in Middle Eastern cultures, and Myrrh is itself a resinous tree.[78] Sweet scented and generating a thick, black smoke, tree resins are associated in many cultures with deep cleansing and with profound prayers. Smoke carries prayers outward into the world. Laurie says that Pine resin was traditionally used as an incense in Ireland during the time when the trees were still abundant there.[79] Interestingly, the word *dé* is both the nominative form of the word for a puff of smoke and the genitive form of the word for god, which suggests to me a possible but unprovable etymological link—incense smoke belongs to the gods.

Resins are the secretions of trees—their equivalent of sweat and tears. They help to heal wounded places on the trunk, so I tend to gather them very, very gently, making sure to take only what has accumulated from older flows of resin and never harvesting down to the bark. I often will use a strip of fallen Birch bark to hold the Spruce and Pine resin I collect with my fingers or with a ritual blade, and then burn bark and resin together when I need to pray for an infusion of the breath of life into the world or for purification.

Pine resin is also a profound medicine for healing the lungs. Its light aromatic molecules, monoterpenes and sesquiterpenes, are warming and aromatic, opening the airways, relaxing the mind, and inviting deep breath. The heavier aromatic molecules, the diterpenes, the sticky molecules that hold the resin together, have a special gift for breaking up sticky phlegm. All of these compounds are topically antimicrobial and inhaling them is a topical treatment for your respiratory tract.

Smoke, of course, contains irritating and potentially harmful particulates, so steam is a better way to administer the medicine. When I was sick with an acute COVID-19 infection, I gathered Pine cones with thick dollops of resin on them and Pine boughs freshly brought down by the wind, along with Alder cones and catkins. I boiled water and then brought the temperature down to steaming and added the cones, branches, and catkins to the water and covered it, keeping the heat on for ten minutes. Then I removed the pot from the heat and placed a towel over my head and the pot and breathed in the steam. When I lived in a yurt in Washington, I would treat respiratory infections in a similar way but would heat the water on the woodstove and then remove it to let it cool before beginning to inhale the steam. Afterward, I would add more water and put the pot of medicine back on the stove so it could infuse the air with healing steam throughout the day. I prefer this method, but alas, had no woodstove when COVID-19 hit me.

Pine is a profoundly solar medicine, gathering sunlight in winter. The Christmas tree and the Christmas wreath are modern echoes of older traditions among northern peoples of bringing evergreen boughs indoors in winter to honor the sun and to fill the home with their scent. In Irish and Scottish cultures, and in those of the insular Celtic peoples, Pine has traditionally been associated with virility and fertility.

In spring, the Pine releases copious yellow pollen. In Chinese medicine, this pollen is a traditional yang tonic. Stephen Harrod Buhner has noted that the pollen in Scots Pine contains a compound identical to human testosterone.[80] Reductionists have argued that the concentration of this molecule is too low to be pharmacologically significant, but human endocrine systems are complex and sensitive things, subject to very subtle influences. I can say that from my own experience and from those of others I have spoken with, the pollens of many Pine species stimulate vitality and libido and increase the production of new muscle tissue in conjunction with exercise in ways that relate directly to testosterone's action in the human body. They don't seem to stimulate hair growth in the way testosterone does and don't seem strong enough to be a substitute for medical testosterone supplementation in people seeking physical changes in their gender presentation. But they definitely increase the felt sense of the primal energies our culture calls masculine.

The presence and the medicine of Pine stirs us to life even in winter.

Safety considerations: None.

Ecological considerations: Prolific where forests have not been felled.

🌿 Psilocybin (*Psilocybe* spp.)

A few winters ago, I was invited to take part in another culture's medicine ceremony. The spirit of the plant we were working with told me that I was welcome to partake in the ceremony but that my people once had a similar ritual of their own. The plant spirit called in my ancestors who showed me a vision of a man in a stone chamber wrapped in furs, playing the bodhrán, while people sat around a fire, singing and passing around a bowl of a purplish liquid I recognized as a tea made from *Psilocybe* mushrooms. Several months later, I found myself standing atop a hill in a ring of Oaks planted by Gwydion Pendderwen, a bard of my tradition who had died young decades ago. I was there praying to understand how to dedicate my life to the living world without courting a similar death. His spirit had been among those who had visited me in the ceremony the winter before.

I had a vision of the queen of the Otherworld standing before me, and then I once again saw a dark stone chamber. This chamber was smaller, the size of one man's tomb, and I saw myself lying there wrapped in a Bear skin, completely still with my hands on my chest, while a woman poured that same mushroom tea into my mouth and then left and sealed the chamber.

The queen told me that Bears spend nine months walking the earth and three months sleeping beneath it, listening to the songs of roots, mycelia, and buried bones. She said that once upon a time, men who were pledged to her did the same—spending the dark months of the year in a continuous dreaming state brought on by being continuously fed bone broth and mushroom tea and the bright months bringing the visions incubated there to life. This is an inversion of the year that followed our conception, when we spent nine months in the womb and three months in this world, learning its ways. She said that this was not possible in the world as it is, but that I should do what I could to follow suit in ways that fit this time and place: making the dark of the year an inward time as best I could, working with small doses of the mushrooms throughout the season and larger doses when I was in need of a more powerful vision and could carve out the time and space.

Erynn Rowan Laurie tells us that the *filidh* used periods of "incubatory darkness" to cultivate states of poetic ecstasy, and she and Timothy White provide evidence that they may have used the *Amanita muscaria* mushroom as well.[81] These rites likely echo Paleolithic practices of descending into caves to communicate with the spirits of animals. In the case of these Stone Age practices, hypoxia, darkness, and the acoustics of the caves likely played a role in inducing the visionary states people entered. Given that humans around the world have worked with mind-altering mushrooms, and other species do too, it is possible that there was a psychedelic element to these early rituals. The oldest human-made object found in Ireland is a Bear bone carved into a tool found in a cave in Clare. The chambers at the heart of the Sidhe, the burial mounds believed to be the home of the Daoine Sidhe, were likely attempts to replicate at least some of these same conditions.

Psilocybe semilanceata is ubiquitous in Irish pastures as Samhain approaches. Nobody knows for certain how long this has been true. The dominant theory in the mycological world is that the mushroom arrived in Ireland from North America sometime in the past two centuries, but this is based on a lack of documentation of the species there prior to 1925. The absence of documentation doesn't necessarily mean the absence of the mushroom. People would have been unlikely to tell outsiders about such a medicine if they did, indeed, work with it. Some theorize that *Psilocybe* mushrooms may have been used in the *teach alais,* the sweathouse. There is only the slightest bit of circumstantial evidence that this may be true, but it is consistent with the visions I was shown, which predated my reading Laurie's work and my reading about the teach alais by several years.

Regardless of whether they were used historically as a ritual medicine outside the places in Mexico where we have information about their traditional use, the many mushrooms of the *Psilocybe* genus make more sense as a visionary medicine for people today than *Amanita muscaria* does. *Amanita muscaria* can be toxic, is hard on the liver, and can easily and disastrously be misidentified. *Psilocybe* mushrooms are far gentler.

Herbalist jim mcdonald says that there are certain plants whose habitat is the places where people live. These plants, such as Dandelion and Plantain, tend to follow the path of civilization's spread and provide safe, gentle, but profound medicine. One could say something similar about *Psilocybe* mushrooms: they love pastures created by people and livestock, with many species favoring grasses whose roots are nourished by Cow and Sheep manure. They are gentler than most other psychedelic medicines, though the journeys they bring you on, especially at high doses, can be quite intense.

I think of them as showing up at civilization's edge as an antidote to civilization's mental poisons. A recent study done in London found that people with moderate depression who were given a regimen of meditation and psilocybin (one of the two primary serotonergic alkaloids in *Psilocybe* mushrooms) in addition to experiencing relief from their depression experienced a decreased willingness to accept the dictates of illegitimate authority and an increased sense of connection to nature. It is worth noting that *Psilocybe semilanceata*'s common name, Liberty

Cap, is connected with its cap's resemblance to the caps worn by French revolutionaries in the late eighteenth century. Whether the mushroom was named for the cap, or the cap was meant to represent the mushroom is a mystery.

Researchers are a bit mystified about the way in which psilocybin relieves depression. Most modern antidepressants work by slowing the reuptake of neurotransmitters to make them last longer. Psilocybin does not. It does act on serotonin and dopamine receptors, but in idiosyncratic ways more similar to those of the brain of a child learning new things or a person from the city brought into the wilderness. Rather than directly relieving the symptoms of depression, it seems to give people a new perspective on what is making them depressed. In part, it does so by stimulating the production of new synapses, just as serotonin itself does.

One-time large doses of psilocybin have proven effective in shifting the anxiety and depression of people who have been diagnosed with terminal illness, when those people are given guidance and a safe setting. Those shifts seem to be permanent, with people still showing positive effects from the treatment six months later. I suspect the shifts would be even more profound if the therapy were administered in a forest instead of a hospital room.

Psilocybe is undoubtedly an Otherworld medicine. It is the fruiting body of a web of connections that runs underground and feeds off the nutrients released by the decay of things that have died. It is no wonder that it facilitates a sense of connection with the living world.

Microdosing with *Psilocybe* mushrooms has been growing in popularity, both as a way of managing depression and as a way of increasing creativity. I have seen it help people accomplish both goals, but I offer several caveats. If you are taking *Psilocybe* mushrooms to address depression but you have been living an unexamined life, you may for a time get more depressed, because the medicine invites you to look at what dwells beneath the surface of your consciousness. But if you do the work of trying to engage the questions the medicine brings to the surface, it will help you find ways of answering those questions that you might not otherwise have imagined. And if you are taking *Psilocybe* because you want to write better advertising jingles for toothpaste, it might help you to do that at first, but it's likely that it will eventually make you begin to question why you are writing stupid songs about toothpaste instead of songs about the things that make you feel alive. If you are taking the mushrooms so you can make more creative arguments to defend your client's oil pipeline, expect some nightmares. Parts of corporate America are infatuated with psychedelic microdosing right about now, but wild medicines are not easily harnessed or safely appropriated for furthering the goals of this civilization. Early results of larger doses of psilocybin in people with treatment-resistant depression point in this direction: in addition to experiencing a remission of their depression, patients in one study reported feeling increased affinity for nature and a decreased willingness to accept authoritarian ideas and stricture.

My preferred method of microdosing is to make an oxymel by filling a jar to the top with dried mushrooms (I personally favor *Psilocybe cubensis*) and macerating them in a combination of two-thirds vinegar and one-third honey. The vinegar, being acidic, helps to extract the psilocybin and psilocyin, which are alkaline, and the honey helps to preserve the preparation. Stored in a cool, dark place, it has a shelf life of about a year in a New England climate. I recommend starting with a dose of three to five drops a day. Once you are used to the way the medicine feels, you can try slightly higher doses, titrating upward, before spending time in the forest or beneath the stars. Five milliliters is about the threshold at which I start to notice visual shifts, but I am a tall man and have worked with the medicine for a long time, so I don't recommend doing anything that requires focused attention after taking more than one milliliter of the oxymel until you know how the medicine works in your particular body.

Microdosing is best done in a quiet place, in dim light or darkness, where you will have an opportunity to be contemplative. This practice can be especially rich to engage in during the time between Samhain and Imbolc.

> **Safety considerations:** Too large a dose will make you vomit, which makes it hard for these mushrooms to cause physical poisoning. As with all psychedelics, great emotional and spiritual caution are advised, especially for those with a personal or family history of psychosis.
>
> **Ecological considerations:** Abundant and easily cultivated.

🌿 Rose (*Rosa* spp.)

There is, perhaps, no scent more evocative than that of a blooming Rose carried on the wind on a summer morning just after a rain. In *Virdarium Umbris*, herbalist and occultist Daniel Schulke writes: "The Soul of the Rose is exalted within the dew on her petals."[82] It is a scent that invites us into an immediate sensual experience of the world around us, seducing us into embodied connection by reminding us of beauty.

Roses engage our senses deeply. The reds, pinks, whites, and yellows of the blossoms draw our eyes and speak of the gradual unfurling of mysteries to those who approach with loving attention. The petals caress our skin, and their medicine soothes raging heat. Their scent opens the heart.

Rose's reputation as an aphrodisiac comes from its simultaneous capacity to soothe us and delight our senses, making us more open to intimacy. But that intimacy need not be with a human lover or partner and need not be sexual in the sense in which our culture tends to use the word; it can be erotic in a broader sense. Eros is the drive for life, vitality, and connection. When we define the erotic in this sense, the definition of an aphrodisiac broadens as well. Aphrodisiacs are those medicines that invite us into deep presence and relation. Absolutely, an aphrodisiac can be a love potion in the conventional sense, but it can just as easily be an herb that invites a despondent spirit to remain in the world. One winter I had a client struggling with deep depression ask his partner to bring him Roses every week and prepare him baths with the petals. The medicine helped him remain alive and engaged during a season in which his senses were often dulled and his heart often slumbering.

The Heart of the Rose is an old Craft name for the womb of the Mother of the World, from which all things emerge. This association of Rose and the Divine Mother was kept alive in Catholic Europe and filtered into syncretic folk religions through Latin America. I frequently work with Roses in my devotional work with the Mother, inviting connection with her by softening and opening my heart, just as I might in meeting a human lover. Sometimes I will bathe with Rose petals in preparation for a ritual with her, sometimes I will anoint myself with Rose water, sometimes I will take a few drops of a Rose tincture or drink Rose tea, sometimes I will place Roses on my altar. All serve to shift my felt sense of myself to make me more receptive to her presence.

The sepals of the Rose form a five-pointed star—a shape also found in the center of the many Rose family fruits. The pentacle they form is a symbol that speaks to the structure of reality in profound ways. It is, of course, famously the shape formed by the stance of Leonardo da Vinci's famous Vitruvian man—facing forward with limbs extended. It is also a representation of an endless flow, kin to the knotwork of medieval and ancient Irish art. These are deep mysteries connected with this shape best learned through direct contemplation of it in a Rose garden.

Then there is Rose's gentle astringency. Many people think of astringents as herbs that dry us out, but in fact they bind together tissue fibers and seal membranes to help them hold in fluids, preventing them from flowing out too rapidly. Rose simultaneously awakens, soothes, and holds the heart. I often give Rose to people who keep sobbing themselves into exhaustion and then as soon as they regain energy begin to sob again. Rose's astringency is mild enough to allow tears to still flow but strong enough to help a person hold onto enough of her own life force to walk through all that grief demands—while the coolness of the petals soothes the heart's burning pain, and the sweetness of the flower reminds the heart of joy.

Magically, that astringency helps to keep my consciousness and attention focused in my heart, to bring a tenderness to all I do. I also work with Rose magically to soften and contain hot, intense emotions that arise during or around the work I am doing, or that are driving the situation I am trying to change. For example, I might use Rose in a spell to try to prevent one person's anger from spilling over into active aggression against another.

But not all of Rose's medicine is tender. Schulke writes:

The Rose stands at the heart of the Garden as the Arbor Inscrutable. As within, her power is also magnified without, she is the running thorns standing as Sentinel of Paradise. . . . The Genius abides in quiet and strength, guarding her perfumed nectars. The essence of her devotion is manifest in her impeccable manner of self-protection, her determination to thrive in adversity, her respect of kindred, her quiet humility as she goes about her work in the shade of trees far taller.[83]

The thorn is as essential a part of the magic and deep medicine of Rose as the blossom. Like Hawthorn, Rose shares beauty and nourishment freely precisely because its thorns establish a boundary that creates a space in which openness is possible. Her body will not be touched without invitation and only then with careful attention. I learned from jim mcdonald that many tenderhearted people need to take on some of Rose's thorniness to establish healthy boundaries, and that giving a person a Rose thorn to carry as a talisman can help to impart that aspect of Rose's way of being to a person who needs it. I think of such a talisman as a somatic cue reminding a person of the quality of sharpness.

Through shifting our sensory experience, Rose helps us to change the patterns we impart on our bodies and on the world.

Safety considerations: None.

Ecological considerations: Prolific in areas where it is wild or introduced and easily cultivated.

ꙮ Rowan (*Sorbus* spp.)

In May, the Rowan is bedecked with white flowers. In August, it is laden with red berries, which will feed the birds well into winter. The berries are astringent and tart with a hint of bitterness. They grow sweeter after the first frost, when they are traditionally harvested and stewed to make jelly. Rowan berries strung together as a necklace are a traditional amulet of protection from hostile magic. During late summer, I gather Rowan berries and place them on all the lintels of my home. In winter, I feed them to the birds.

Color is important in understanding the tree's traditional associations. According to Fayerie traditionalist and spiritual ecologist Robin Artisson, red in Celtic cultures is the color of life and power in this world, associated with the blood of the living, and white is the color of the Otherworld, associated with the white bones of the dead.[84] Both the Hawthorn and the Rowan have white flowers, which give way to red berries. The Hawthorn, however, is more a protector of the Otherworld whose influence crosses over into this one, while the Rowan is associated with protecting the living from baleful Otherworld influences. The transition from white to red suggests a certain regulation of the flow of power from the Otherworld into this one.

The name Rowan is related to the Norse word *rune* and the Sanskrit word *runa*, which means "magician." The wood is still used in Icelandic magic for carving rune spells, especially spells of protection, and in Scotland to make protective crosses bound together with red thread. The cross predates Christianity as an important symbol in Irish and Scottish cultures, most likely a solar symbol originally, though it has accrued layers of Christian meaning over the centuries as well.

Traditionally, in both Ireland and Scotland, Rowan wood fires were used to bless and protect cattle in May while denizens of the Otherworld were about causing mischief, and some livestock were given collars of Rowan wood. Cattle were the primary form of wealth among Gaelic peoples before English laws and customs were imposed on them in the seventeenth century.[85] As with other trees, if you are going to work with Rowan wood, I strongly suggest either using only fallen branches or finding a place where a tree is being felled by someone for other reasons and asking the person felling it for some of the wood. If doing the latter, if at all possible, make offerings of honey, whiskey, and milk to the tree before it is felled.

In some areas, people believe that Rowan will never be struck by lightning—an interesting contrast with the Oak, which is said to draw lightning and survive its strike. The Norse associate the Oak with Thor and the Rowan with Thor's wife, Sif. The Rowan is also said to have saved Thor's life when he grasped a Rowan growing over a rushing stream that had swept him away. If you find your life is prone to sudden disaster coming like a bolt from the sky, I suggest sitting with the Rowan each day and asking how you can learn to have the lightning pass you by.

In Irish, the tree is called *caorthann*, derived from *caor*, a word that means both "berry" and "flame." It is related to the letter *luis* in the ancient Irish Ogham alphabet, which is associated with "the luster of the eye" (similar to the brightness of the eyes associated with healthy Shen in Chinese medicine), the fire of inspiration of the goddess Brighid, and drawing magic from the Otherworld to sustain and protect life in this world. Similar associations among the Brythonic peoples of Wales and England led to its naming as the Quickening Tree, from the Old English *cwicu*, reaching back to the Proto-Indo-European root word *gʷihₜwós*, meaning "alive."[86]

Old Irish texts speak of one particular Rowan that grew from a seed accidentally planted by the the Tuath Dé after they arrived from the Land of Promise to the North. As Lady Gregory relates the story:

The provision the [Tuath Dé] had brought with them from the Land of Promise was crimson nuts [which Rowan and White suggest may refer to the red and white psychotropic mushroom *Amanita muscaria*, an important ritual medicine of many northern peoples], and apples, and sweet-smelling rowan berries. And as they were passing through the district of

Ui Fiachrath by the Muaidh, a berry of the rowan berries fell from them, and a tree grew up from it. And there was virtue in its berries, and no sickness or disease would ever come on any person that would eat them, and those that would eat them would feel the liveliness of wine and the satisfaction of mead in them, and any old person of a hundred years that would eat them would go back to be young again, and any young girl that would eat them would grow to a flower of beauty.[87]

Similarly, Greek myth tells us that the Rowan was turned red by blood falling from the body of a great Eagle as he flew above after rescuing the cup that bore the restorative nectar of the gods after it was stolen by evil spirits. Making a syrup of Rowan berries in honey or a Rowan berry mead or cordial can be a beautiful way of connecting with this aspect of the tree's magic. Mulling spices will make a good addition. In moments that you need to connect with what nourishes the red blood of life, focus on the intent and feeling of restoration, visualize the source of the water that nourishes you and the land where you live, and take a sip. Then ask to flower with beauty and to bring forth the fruit of the true work of the being you are.

> **Safety considerations:** If you plan to ingest the berries, cook or dry them first. The raw berries contain parasorbic acid, which is very irritating to the digestive tract but is converted to harmless sorbic acid by hydrolyzation.
>
> **Ecological status:** Abundant in its traditional European homeland and the areas where it has become naturalized in North America.

🌿 Solomon's Seal *(Polygonatum bifolium)*

Solomon's Seal grows from rich forest soils, its stem making a graceful arc that bends back toward the ground. A pair of small white flowers grow beneath each pair of leaves along the stem, becoming blue berries in late summer. Beneath the ground, a bone-white root grows, each year producing a new joint.

The medicine of Solomon's Seal's root is sweet, nourishing, and moistening. It contains allantoin, a compound that aids in the regrowth of skin, bone, and fascia, but for reasons not yet fully known to our science, it has an "intelligence" that prevents those tissues from growing back too rapidly. This is unlike Comfrey (*Symphytum* spp.), the other primary allantoin-rich plant, which can cause a bone to regrow too quickly in the wrong position or cause skin to regrow so quickly over a wound that it can seal in infection. Some of this may be related to the presence of certain lectins in Solomon's Seal that appear to help regulate both apoptosis (natural cell death) and autophagy (the elimination of dead and unhealthy cells). The lectins in a Chinese relative of Solomon's Seal are being investigated as potential novel agents in treating skin cancers.

Like most sweet roots, Solomon's Seal also has an ability to aid in the generation of healthy new fluids. In Taoist and ayurvedic medicine, the Chinese and Indian varieties of Solomon's Seal have strong reputations as fertility medicines because of their ability to help increase generation of sexual fluids. Its polysaccharides help to stimulate the production of mucus to lubricate the respiratory and digestive tracts, as well as soothing inflammation there. When I was dealing with acute COVD-19, my lungs felt like they were made of hot, dry leather, and Solomon's Seal helped restore moisture and pliability to the tissues. Interestingly, I once heard jim mcdonald use a similar analogy to describe the fascia of people who need Solomon's Seal. Solomon's Seal appears to have a strong affinity for synovial fluid, which lubricates our fascia—an insight Matthew Wood brought forward a few decades ago. A few drops will quickly increase mobility in fascial tissues of all kinds. This may also be one of the reasons I found it so helpful when I was dealing with COVID. The pleura which surround the lungs are fascia, and pleuritis, inflammation of that pleural fascial tissue is a common symptom of COVID and other respiratory illnesses. For this purpose, Solomon's Seal combines well with Mullein and Pleurisy Root (*Asclepias tuberosa*), also known as Butterfly Weed. We also have fascial tissue around the heart—the pericardium. Interestingly, both Solomon's Seal and Pleurisy Root have shared affinities for the lungs, heart, and joints.

The roots of many of Solomon's Seal's Asparagus family kin—such as False Solomon's Seal (*Smilacina racemosa*), Shatavari (*Asparagus racemose*), and Asparagus (*Asparagus officianalis*)—share these moistening properties, and Shatavari and Asparagus root make good, sustainable substitutes for Solomon's Seal when the goal is to generate new fluids. Culpepper noted that the root of Asparagus "doth moisten the sinews"— a long-forgotten virtue that this common garden vegetable shares with its cousins.[88] I am not fully convinced that all of these *Asparagaceae* plants share Solomon's Seal's gifts for aiding healthy growth of bones, fascia, and epithelial tissues, however. Interestingly, the tinctures of all of these roots seem to work as well in this regard as their decoctions, despite the fact that polysaccharides are water soluble but not easily alcohol soluble. For this reason, however, I do suggest shaking up the tinctures before taking them since sometimes some of the polysaccharides may precipitate out and fall to the bottom of the bottle or jar.

I have found Solomon's Seal to be especially helpful with the musculoskeletal issues of aging dogs. I tend to give them small doses of the tincture diluted in water. Solomon's Seal helped my Siberian Husky greatly with her arthritis during the final years of her life. And I have twice used Solomon's Seal together with Mullein root to restore mobility for an elderly Dachshund after falls exacerbated old spinal injuries.

Native root doctor Tis Mal Crow writes that his people learned that Solomon's Seal is also healing to the gut from watching Wolves:

The Muskogee people learned about Solomon's Seal from the Wolf. By observing animals in the wild and studying what plants, roots, and barks they used for food and medicine, the Muskogee people learned about many uses for plants from the different animals that used them. The Wolf was observed using the root of Solomon's Seal whenever he had stomach problems. If the Wolf had eaten too much or had eaten old meat or something hard to digest, he would dig and eat the roots. The Muskogee refer to Solomon's Seal as a Wolf Medicine. I have also heard that the German name for Solomon's Seal translates to "Wolf's Milk."[89]

Part of this is likely due to the reduction of inflammation in the epithelial tissues of the gut and the production of new mucus to soothe the gut lining. But based on observing the way in which Solomon's Seal helped people who had been taking antibiotics recover their digestive health, Crow theorized that the plant might also be helping to restore the gut microbiome. Chinese researchers confirmed in 2018 that Chinese Fragrant Solomon's Seal root (*Polygonatum odoratum*) does in fact improve the health of rodent gut microbiomes, both helping healthy bacteria grow and reducing unhealthy bacteria.[90] Research is proceeding into the possible use of the medicine to aid in conditions related to gut dysbiosis, including diabetes and obesity. For this purpose, it is best to eat a bit of the fresh root with some dirt still on it, next best to chew or decoct the dried root. Matthew Wood once told me that Tis Mal Crow advised people who have had appendectomies to take a pinch of Solomon's Seal root in bone broth each day. We now know that the appendix holds elements of our gut microbiome in reserve to help repopulate the gut after the gut flora have been wiped out.

Matthew Wood speaks of the more esoteric meaning of Solomon's Seal being a Wolf medicine:

The Wolf Medicines usually have a ninety-degree angle in their construction, indicating an affinity for making profound changes or turns in life. They help bring a person to a transformative place, or help them go through a change, or help them adapt to a change that has already occurred. The ninety-degree angle represents joints in the organism and key-joints in the path of life.[91]

Wood associates this with aligning with destiny, which he defines as "a fork in the road where we have the opportunity to associate ourselves with something new."[92] When engaged in this way, I think of Solomon's Seal as smoothing the motion of the spirit in the same way that it smooths the motion of the body. Interestingly, something of this sense is captured in the Anglo-Saxon name for the plant, *hlædder-wyrt,* which translates literally to "ladder wort" and is a reference to Jacob's ladder to heaven.[93] Taoist medicine speaks of destiny as the river that flows from the reservoir of our ancestral inheritance, the waters of the kidneys, guided by the stars under which we are born and under which we live. Due to its moist, nourishing nature, Solomon's Seal is a kidney yin tonic that helps that river flow smoothly. In times of disruption, it combines well with Devil's Club (*Oplopanax horridus*) to bring protection and new growth in the wake of that disruption and Rose (*Rosa* spp.) to bring some sweetness to the heart.

Solomon's Seal brings together the earth element's gifts of nourishment and structure with the water element's gift of flow. Often the addition of a bit of fire in the form of a warming plant like Ginger (*Zingiber officanalis*), Devil's Club, or Calamus (*Acorus* spp.) will help set the flow in motion. Damiana (*Turnera diffusa*) serves especially well here as an herb that both gets the blood flowing and restores pleasure in movement. Lobelia (*Lobelia inflata*) and Black Cohosh (*Cimicifuga racemosa*) help dilate blood vessels and reduce, respectively, tension and inflammation in the muscles, making then nice adjuncts to Solomon's Seal. Together with these allies, Solomon's Seal brings grace to the ways we move.

> **Safety considerations:** Solomon's Seal root contains very low levels of cardiac glycosides. In some cases this can be beneficial: Matthew Wood likes to use Solomon's Seal and Hawthorn (*Crataegus* spp.) together as a heart tonic.[94] However, caution is required when giving this medicine to someone who is taking a cardiac glycoside medication such as digoxin for congestive heart failure. The leaf and the berries are considered toxic by many; however, both Indigenous people and rural white Scots-Irish people in several parts of North America have traditionally used the leaf for medicine. I cannot personally attest to the safety of any part but the root.

Ecological considerations: Solomon's Seal is facing overharvesting in many parts of North America. It can, however, be fairly easily cultivated, though you will have to wait seven years or so for the root to be ready for harvest. A few herb farms are growing the plant and selling the root; it's best to get it from them. In some soils, like those in New England and the Upper Midwest, because Solomon's Seal propagates by runner, you can trace the runner as it goes underground between plants, cut the middle section, and replant both ends, and the plant will continue to thrive—a technique taught by jim mcdonald. However, Laura Quesinberry, whose family has many generations of experience working with Solomon's Seal in Appalachia, says that this technique will not work with the plants that grow in the South.

✻ Trillium (*Trillium erectum*)

Trillium blossoms bright red in the forests of New England right after the snows have receded, when the sun is bright enough to warm the soil but the nights are still cold. Wake Robin is one of its common names in some places, signaling the relationship of its blooming with the Robin's return.

The flower's three petals supported by three sepals remind me of the structure of the pelvic bones and the ligaments that connect them. Birth Root is another name for Trillium because if its ability to tone the pelvis in preparation for childbirth. Its crimson petals also suggest its capacity to stop uterine hemorrhage. It was also historically used to check the pulmonary bleeding associated with tuberculosis.

Today, Trillium is too rare in New England to justify harvest under all but the rarest of circumstances. It is a medicine to be experienced primarily through its presence. To bring its presence into another time and place, use a flower essence. The essence is best made from a single flower placed in a crystal bowl of water in the early morning, picked with twigs without touching it with your hands or damaging any other part of the plant. Place the bowl in sunlight until at least noon, then combine the water with an equal part of brandy to preserve it. Kate Gilday of Woodland Essence describes the flower essence of Red Trillium as providing "tender yet strong support during times of birth, death and re-birth."[95] This resonates strongly with my own sense of the presence of the plant, captured in a poem the Trillium gave me just before Bealtaine many years ago:

> *Deep crimson blossoms*
> *recall blood*
> *and the taste of iron,*
>
> *spray of stars*
> *in the center*
> *guide you in*
>
> *to the caress*
> *of petals*
>
> *that draw you*
> *down to*
> *darkness.*
>
> *Blooming*
> *in the moments*
> *before spring*
> *has decided*
> *whether*
> *to remain,*
>
> *Our Lady of the Forest*
> *draws no distinction*
> *between birth*
> *and death.*

Whichever passage
you choose
she will hold you
through the night

then deliver you
to the spring morning,

Stillborn
or drawing
your first breath.

Safety considerations: For ecological reasons, I do not advocate working with the physiological medicine of this plant, but it is generally considered safe. If you do choose to work with this plant during pregnancy, do so only under the supervision of a midwife familiar with this medicine.

Ecological considerations: This plant depends on very particular mycorrhizal relationships to thrive, which are next to impossible to replicate outside its natural environment. It also takes many years for its root to reach the size of a Bumble Bee. The only way to ethically harvest this flower and its root, which is the source of its physiological medicine, is to do so from places that are about to be bulldozed or clear-cut. Otherwise, it is best to work with the flower essence.

🌿 Wormwood (*Artemisia absinthium*)

Wormwood is a potent herb that helps to reawaken our memory of who we are. Modern conceptions of the herb tend to revolve around its use in treating parasitic infections—from malaria to pinworms—but physical parasites are not the only kind of "pernicious external influence" (to borrow a term from Chinese medicine) that Wormwood can help us drive out.

Our contemporary culture is one of the few that does not speak of possession as a source of illness. If we understand possession to mean the invasion of our own being by another consciousness that doesn't have our best interest in mind, a parasite of consciousness, and if we realize that such a being doesn't have to have a humanlike form, we can see how we all give over a degree of mental and emotional control to disembodied forces. Is there a real difference between writing a document that gives a thought-form and a name to a corporation or a government and performing incantations and drawing sigils to summon angels and demons—especially when people then make decisions that prioritize the needs, desires, and survival of that entity over their own values and well-being in exchange for money or protection? I would contend that as a culture, we do not speak of possession not because it is rare but because it is ubiquitous.

The late Dale Pendell contended that the Wormwood's old Saxon name *wermod,* from which the word *vermouth* is also derived, meant "defend the mind."[96] He was likely drawing on the work of an early twentieth-century philologist, Ernest Weekley, who theorized that wermod was a compound word whose components meant "man" (*wer*) and "courage" (*mod*).

The great seventeenth-century herbalist and astrologer Nicholas Culpeper said that his understanding and description of Wormwood contained the key to understanding his entire approach to medicine. Because of its profound heat and its tendency to grow near forges, Culpeper ascribed Wormwood's rulership to Mars and asserted that, in relation to humanity, Mars's "only desire is [that] they should know themselves."[97]

In the Greek-derived medicine that Culpeper studied and practiced, heat is identified with the life force and cold is seen as breaking down a being's identity. The profound heat of Wormwood helps in reasserting that identity.

A generation earlier, Shakespeare seems to have tapped into this same aspect of Wormwood's medicine when he describes the Faerie King Oberon using the herb, which he calls "Dian's bud," to break the spell he had cast on his queen, Titania, which had caused her to fall in love with an ass. Giving the remedy, Oberon said:

> *Be as thou wast wont to be*
> *See as thou wast wont to see:*
> *Dian's bud o'er Cupid's flower*
> *Hath such force and blessed power.*
> *Now, my Titania, wake you, my sweet queen.*

It is worth noting here that Matthew Wood says that Wormwood is an herb for someone who "wakes in a convulsion or a trance"—its heat stimulates the nervous system to rouse consciousness.[98] Drawing on that usage, I frequently give drop doses of this herb to people experiencing intense nightmares and to people experiencing dissociation. In the latter case, I like to combine it with Calamus. In both cases, I combine it with Wood Betony (*Stachys betonica*), an herb that helps people anchor more deeply in their bodies in the present time and space.

There is some interesting cultural blending at play here that suggests some ancient truths. The character of Titania is clearly based on the cultural memory of Celtic Faerie queens, who embodied the spirit of the living land, before they were tamed and diminished in the collective imagination as they would be in the Victorian era. Her name, however, is believed to be a variation on that of Diana, Roman goddess of the moon and the hunt, who, in turn, was a syncretized version of the Greek Artemis, who, like Pan, arose from the trace memory of wild spirits who people had known since the Paleolithic. Artemis gives her name to *Artemisia*, the genus of plants to which Wormwood belongs (which Shakespeare references by naming it Dian's bud). So, the medicine that cures Titania of her delusion and amnesia is, in fact, an herb that embodies her essence.

Titania, is, of course, portrayed as lusty and free, while Artemis and Diana are traditionally viewed as virginal. There is not, however, as strong a disconnect here as one might think at first. As German religious scholar Julia Iwersen writes: "The Greek Artemis is clearly the heiress of the Mistress of the Animals, but her wildness was acceptable in a patriarchal culture only if it was understood that she was not like other women. Thus she was superficially bereft of her female sexuality."[99]

In a classical Athenian cultural framework, that "female sexuality" would have been understood as something that needed to be controlled and harnessed for the purposes of reproduction. Susun Weed and others have suggested that in such a context, "virginity" can be understood to mean being outside masculine control rather than necessarily implying chastity.

Certainly, this is the sense that I get from my own encounters with Artemis and her herbs. At one level, we can understand Wormwood and its cousin, Mugwort, which Culpeper saw as ruled by Venus,[100] as herbs of the wild feminine outside masculine control. On another level, as herbs that replace externally imposed concepts of identity with the identity that arises organically from within, they tend to break down our cultural categories of gender, and they frequently show up to help when I am working with people who in one way or another are struggling with the cultural and social constraints connected with the gender they were assigned at birth. Every time I work with any of the plants associated with Artemis, I hear a voice saying, "My gender is not feminine; it is wild."

This points to another important aspect of Wormwood's medicine. Matthew Wood writes that Wormwood "is suited to people who have been brutalized by the reverses of life, including poverty and abuse," especially when they are dealing with "chronic depression, lack of affect, deadness, hopelessness."[101] In other words, it is an herb that is helpful when oppression causes depression by suppressing someone's sense of self and power.

I learned from Wood to give just one or two drops of Wormwood a week when someone is in that kind of flat, lifeless depression, because he warns that more than that can bring on further depression. My own sense here is that a tiny bit of Wormwood reawakens consciousness, but more of it brings suppressed things to consciousness.

When I am working with someone who is feeling gray and lifeless, I give one drop of Wormwood a week and work with drop doses of *Angelica* or Damiana in between those treatments.

I will give Wormwood more frequently when a person is actively working to reintegrate buried aspects of his consciousness, and in those cases, I give it in combination with Black Cohosh and Solomon's Seal or Shatavari. This combination is also indicated for the frequently co-occurring stiffness and rheumatic pain that arise from long-term body armoring.

Curiously, at highly concentrated doses, when distilled with other herbs to make absinthe, Wormwood has a somewhat opposite effect: it brings a fluid bliss to the body and changes the perception of light, giving it a shimmering, fluid quality as well. True absinthe is sadly illegal to sell in the United States because of concerns about its liver toxicity—which are largely based on old French propaganda about the drink. Absinthe was historically the drink of choice of bohemians and war veterans in France, two groups of people who drank heavily and acted strangely and many of whom developed liver disease. Thujone, the major psychotropic compound in Wormwood (as in Yarrow, Mugwort, and Cedar) can, indeed, be toxic to the liver. But in recent years, medical historians have concluded that those who died from drinking too much absinthe most likely died not of thujone poisoning but of alcohol-induced liver damage, though likely the combination of the two imbibed in large quantities and with great frequency made them die somewhat faster than other alcohol addicts. However, there is little justification for the idea that absinthe is harmful in moderation.

The first time I had absinthe was the only time I briefly met Dale Pendell. He was teaching a workshop about absinthe and passed out samples during class. After the class, I was waiting in line to ask him a question, and the pitcher and paper cups came up and down the long line many times, and I partook each time. The workshop was on a beautifully landscaped college campus, and when I left the building, I found myself standing on a little wooden bridge over a pond with Water Lilies. As I looked at the water, it shimmered with exactly the quality of light Monet portrayed in his famous painting of a similar scene. It dawned on me that Wormwood taught Monet, who loved absinthe, that way of seeing light.

A few years later, a friend shared some beautiful absinthe with me during a conference in Alberta in late summer. When I walked outside a little while later, I saw the aurora borealis, a curtain of green light across the sky that was exactly the same color as the absinthe: the uncannily iridescent hue that gives absinthe the name *la fée verte*—the green fairy.

This dual nature of Wormwood—the ability to bring someone back more fully into this world or to help someone access a way of seeing more like that of the Otherworld—is a quality it shares with its cousin Mugwort (*Artemisia vulgaris*), so called because of its popularity as an herb in beer before the laws replacing it with Hops spoiled everyone's fun. Mugwort is famous as an herb for vivid dreaming, but I learned from Matthew Wood that it can also be an herb for helping someone who is too much in the Otherworld be more grounded in this one. I have found it especially helpful for artists, writers, and musicians who find that Cannabis inspires them to see things in new ways and gets their ideas flowing but also limits their follow-through in actually creating new work. I have them mix a bit of Mugwort with their Cannabis, and all report excellent results.

> **Safety considerations:** Large doses can irritate the digestion and theoretically may cause liver damage, small doses are very safe.
>
> **Ecological considerations:** Prolific in the wild and easily cultivated.

> It is a strange and treacherous excavation,
> the archaeology of the memory in our blood
> that's older than our bones
>
> Sometimes a wound or a scar is the entry point.
> but you must not get stuck there,
> in the hot and stagnant
> > festering pools that form,

or beneath them
in the frenzied, hungry wailing
that becomes the storm
that drives the poison
                    to the surface.

You must dig deeper,
deep enough to see the stars at noon
and there you will hear
a voice in the darkness

giving the stones their names,
singing forests into being,
laying the first notes of the music
that was supposed to call water and earth
into the form of a body
that would shape your ancestors' breath
into a song that could wake
the dead within us.

The music is not lost.
Yours is just to match the singer's rhythm and pitch,
and remember the next note and the next,
until at last you play your movement of the symphony
into resolution

and a voice to come
begins to harmonize with yours
as yours falls into silence
and the music takes and shapes
                    another instrument
and summons another world.

EPILOGUE

Awakening

In the fairy tale, a wicked queen uses poison to put Sleeping Beauty (Aurora) into a deep slumber. While she sleeps, the castle crumbles, as vines and briars climb over its walls.

We have been living that story in reverse. Civilization's spell has caused us to forget who we are. And while our spirits have slumbered, concrete and pavement have replaced the soft forest floor.

But, like Sleeping Beauty, we are awakened by tenderness: by the gentle touch of the living world on our senses.

Humans evolved in forests and savannahs. Our senses and our sensory processing evolved to favor subtle information about the bodies and presence of people, animals, and plants. When we find comfort in the scent of the skin of someone we love, the night chorus of frogs, the sound of leaves rustling in the wind, we are experiencing echoes of what it meant for our ancestors to live in a world they experienced as alive and always speaking to them.

*Our nervous and endocrine systems evolved to respond
to chemical signals from plants that arrived in the
air our ancestors breathed, the water they drank, the
brush of leaf and petal against skin. We feel it still
when the wind brings us the scent of Cottonwood
in springtime, when we walk among Cedars after a
summer rainstorm, when we breathe in the sweet,
pungent perfume of fallen Apples among fallen leaves
in autumn, when we breathe in the scent of Pine and
Fir in the snowy forest.*

*And as we come to our senses, the walls of the fortress
that imprisoned us crumble, and briars grow from
its cracked foundation, bringing sweet Blackberries
warmed in the summer sun to nourish us.*

We rejoin our wild kin, home again at last.

And together we remake the world.

Notes

INTRODUCTION.
BEYOND THE WALLS OF PERCEPTION

1. Buhner, *The Secret Teachings of Plants*, 134.

CHAPTER 1.
LIVING MEDICINE, LIVING MAGIC

1. Leopold and Leopold, *Round River*.
2. Federici, "In Praise of the Dancing Body."
3. Federici, "In Praise of the Dancing Body."
4. Reich, *Ether, God, Devil and Cosmic Superimposition*, 54.
5. Masé, *The Wild Medicine Solution*, 79.
6. Wood, *Vitalism*, 18.
7. Reich, *Ether, God, Devil and Cosmic Superimposition*, 16.

CHAPTER 2.
THE OTHERWORLD WELL

1. Scallon, "Collection of Irish Song Lyrics."
2. Moriarty, *Invoking Ireland*, 41.
3. Artisson, *An Carow Gwyn*, 41.
4. Mac Coitir and D'Arcy, *Ireland's Animals*.
5. Moriarty, *Dreamtime*, 21.

CHAPTER 3.
THE THREE CAULDRONS

1. Laurie, "The Cauldron of Poesy."
2. Laurie, "The Cauldron of Poesy."
3. Dharmananda, "Kidney Essence and the Human Body."
4. Reich, *Ether, God, Devil and Cosmic Superimposition*, 16.
5. Artisson, *An Carow Gwyn*, 260.
6. Hedley, "The Way We Are Designed."
7. Dharmananda, "Kidney Essence and the Human Body."
8. Laurie, "The Cauldron of Poesy."
9. Laurie, "The Cauldron of Poesy."
10. Gantz, *Early Irish Myths and Saga*, 112.
11. Yeats, "The Song of Wandering Aengus."

CHAPTER 4.
MAD, DEAD, OR A POET

1. Heaney, *Sweeney Astray*, 43–44.
2. Moriarty, "Seeking to Walk Beautifully on the Earth."
3. Reich, *The Function of the Orgasm*, 115.
4. Reich, *The Function of the Orgasm*.
5. mcdonald, "Herbal Properties & Actions . . ."
6. Reich, *The Function of the Orgasm*, 146.
7. Reich, *The Function of the Orgasm*, 7.
8. Lifton and Falk, *Indefensible Weapons*.
9. Macy and Brown, *Coming Back to Life*.

CHAPTER 5.
THE SILVER BRANCH

1. Buhner, *Plant Intelligence and the Imaginal Realm*, 199.
2. Buhner, *Plant Intelligence and the Imaginal Realm*, 211.
3. Moriarty, *Dreamtime;* and *Invoking Ireland*.
4. Magan, *Thirty-Two Words for Field*, 33.
5. Moriarty, *Invoking Ireland*, 199.
6. Loughlin, "Gods and Spirits."

7. Murphy, *Finn and the Salmon of Knowledge.*

8. Artisson, *An Carow Gwyn,* 60.

9. Bohbot et al., "Role of the Parahippocampal Cortex."

10. Bohbot et al., "Role of the Parahippocampal Cortex."

11. Carhart-Harris et al., "Neural Correlates of the LSD Experience."

12. Carhart-Harris et al., "Psilocybin for Treatment-Resistant Depression."

13. Leary and Wilson, "How to Wash a Brain," in Leary, *Neuropolitique,* 135.

14. Leary and Wilson, "How to Wash a Brain," 88–89.

15. Leary and Wilson, "How to Wash a Brain," 79.

16. Foucault, *The Birth of the Clinic,* xix.

17. Schiffman, "Psilocybin."

18. Foucault, *The Birth of the Clinic,* 172.

19. Bromwich, "The Capital That Ate Wellness."

20. Roseman, Nutt, and Carhart-Harris, "Quality of Acute Psychedelic Experience."

21. Buhner, *Plant Intelligence and the Imaginal Realm,* 243–464; and Frank, Grinspoon, and Walker, "Intelligence as a Planetary Scale Process."

22. Nayak and Griffiths, "A Single Belief-Changing Psychedelic Experience."

23. Lyons and Carhart-Harris, "Increased Nature Relatedness."

24. Ramos, "The Concepts of Ideology, Hegemony."

25. Buhner, *The Secret Teachings of Plants.*

26. O'Donoghue, *Courting the Wild Queen,* 50.

27. Sheldrake, *Entangled Life,* 51–55.

28. Bedi, Hyman, and de Wit, "Is Ecstasy an 'Empathogen'?"

29. Scahill and Anderson, "Is Ecstasy an Empathogen?"

30. Holze et al., "Distinct Acute Effects of LSD."

31. Lyons and Carhart-Harris, "Increased Nature Relatedness."

32. Nayak and Griffiths, "A Single Belief-Changing Psychedelic Experience."

33. Aaron et al., "Whole Blood Serotonin Levels"; and Shalev and Uzefovsky, "Empathic Disequilibrium."

34. Savarese, "I Object."

35. Dōgen, *Moon in a Dewdrop.*

CHAPTER 6.
ROOTING IN THE LIVING WORLD

1. Buhner, *Secret Teachings of Plants,* 139.

2. Moriarty, *Invoking Ireland,* 57, 61.

3. Benavidez, personal communication.

4. Hedley, "The Way We Are Designed."

CHAPTER 7.
THE WHEEL OF THE YEAR

1. Magan, *Thirty-Two Words for Field,* 11.

2. Artisson, *The Flaming Circle.*

3. Artisson, *The Flaming Circle.*

4. Magan, *Thirty-Two Words for Field,* 33.

5. Jensen, *Listening to the Land,* 310.

6. Heaney, "Requiem for the Croppies," 24.

PLANT AND FUNGAL ALLIES:
PROFILES OF WILD KIN

1. Laurie, *Ogam,* 67.

2. Electronic Dictionary of the Irish Language, s.v. "airech."

3. Electronic Dictionary of the Irish Language, s.v. "dín cridi"; and Laurie, *Ogam,* 67.

4. Hardin, "Alder."

5. Hardin, "Alder."

6. Kvilhaug, *The Seed of Yggdrasill,* 529.

7. Thoreau, "Wild Apples."

8. Tauring, *Runes.*

9. Tauring, *Runes.*

10. Wood, *The Earthwise Herbal: A Complete Guide to Old World Medicinal Plants,* 139.

11. Cook, "Cimicifuga Racemosa."

12. Cook, "Cimicifuga Racemosa."

13. Cook, "Cimicifuga Racemosa."

14. Tozzi, "Does Fascia Hold Memories?"

15. Dimech, "Dynamics of the Occulted Body."

16. Mac Coitir and Langrishe, *Ireland's Trees,* 104.

17. Laurie, *Ogam,* 115.

18. Mac Coitir and Langrishe, *Ireland's Trees,* 106.

19. Daimler, *The Morrigan,* 4.

20. Kuhn, National Women's Hall of Fame.

21. Ren et al., "The Origins of Cannabis Smoking"; and Arie, Rosen, and Namdar, "Cannabis and Frankincense."

22. Pendell and Snyder, *Pharmako Poeia.*

23. Duvall, "A Brief Agricultural History."

24. Zuardi, "History of Cannabis."

25. Zuardi, "History of Cannabis."

26. Ellingwood, *American Materia Medica.*

27. Boericke, "Cannabis Indica, Hashish."

28. Mann, "How San Francisco's HIV/AIDS Warriors Paved the Way."

29. Pellati et al., "*Cannabis Sativa* L. and Nonpsychoactive Cannabinoids."

30. Di Marzo and Piscitelli, "The Endocannabinoid System."

31. Kozela et al., "Cannabinoids Δ9-Tetrahydrocannabinol."

32. Yirmiya, Rimmerman, and Reshef, "Depression as a Microglial Disease"; and Ellingwood, *American Materia Medica.*

33. Hill et al., "Functional Interactions."

34. Senst and Bains, "Neuromodulators, Stress and Plasticity."

35. Di Tomso, Beltramo, and Piomelli, "Brain Cannabinoids in Chocolate."

36. Russo, "Cannabinoids in the Management of Pain."

37. Sulak, "How to Stimulate the Endocannabinoid System."

38. Bensky et al., *Chinese Herbal Medicine,* 120.

39. Russo, "Cannabinoids in the Management of Pain."

40. Prud'homme, Cata, and Jutras-Aswad, "Cannabidiol as an Intervention for Addictive Behaviors"; and Pelatti et al., "*Cannabis Sativa* L. and Nonpsychoactive Cannabinoids."

41. Russo, "Cannabinoids in the Management of Difficult to Treat Pain"; Ko et al., "Medical Cannabis,"; Philpott, O'Brien, and McDougall, "Attenuation of Early Phase Inflammation"; and Vučković et al., "Cannabinoids and Pain"; and Vučković et al., "Cannabinoids and Pain."

42. Bergamaschi et al., "Cannabidiol Reduces the Anxiety."

43. Crippa et al., "Effects of Cannabidiol (CBD)."

44. Lee et al. "Cannabidiol Regulation of Emotion"; and Shannon and Ophila-Lehman, "Effectiveness of Cannabidiol Oil."

45. Lee et al., "Cannabidiol Regulation of Emotion."

46. Bossong et al., "Acute Effects of Δ9-Tetrahydrocannabinol (THC)."

47. Temple, "Here It Is!"

48. Weizmann et al., "Cannabis Analgesia in Chronic Neuropathic Pain."

49. Felter and Lloyd, "Dracontium.—Skunk-Cabbage."

50. Buhner, "SARS-CoV-2 Protocol."

51. Cook, "Symplocarpus Foetidus." 1869b

52. Buhner, "SARS-CoV-2 Protocol."

53. Wood, *The Earthwise Herbal*, 302.

54. Wood, *The Earthwise Herbal*, 304.

55. Wood, *The Earthwise Herbal*, 304.

56. Edwards, *Opening Our Wild Hearts*, 217.

57. Wood, *The Book of Herbal Wisdom*, 201.

58. Lenihan and Green, *Meeting the Other Crowd*.

59. Wood, *The Earthwise Herbal*, 211.

60. Frances, "Crataegus."

61. Woodland Essence, website.

62. Benavidez, *Victor Anderson*, 26.

63. Culpepper, *The Complete Herbal*, 124.

64. Culpepper, *The Complete Herbal*, 124.

65. Cockayne, *Leechdoms, Wortcunning and Starcraft*, 175–76.

66. Mac Coitir and Langrishe, *Ireland's Wild Plants*, 240.

67. Mac Coitir and Langrishe, *Ireland's Wild Plants*, 58.

68. Mac Coitir and Langrishe, *Ireland's Wild Plants*, 59.

69. Mac Coitir and Langrishe, *Ireland's Wild Plants*, 59.

70. Keaney, "Bold Fenian Men."

71. Laurie, *Ogam*, 86.

72. Mac Coitir and Langrishe, *Ireland's Trees*, 59–60.

73. Benavidez, *Victor H. Anderson*, 52.

74. Mac Coitir and Langrishe, *Ireland's Trees*, 114–19.

75. Laurie, *Ogam*, 123.

76. Artisson, *An Carow Gwyn*, 65.

77. Benavidez, *Victor Anderson*, 26.

78. Mac Coitir and Langrishe, *Ireland's Trees*, 28–33.

79. Laurie, *Ogam*, 123.

80. Buhner, *Vital Man*, 110–13.

81. Laurie and White, "Speckled Snake, Brother of Birch."

82. Schulke, *Viridarium Umbris*, 36.

83. Schulke, *Viridarium Umbris*, 36.

84. Artisson, *An Carow Gwyn*, 264.

85. Mac Coitir and Langrishe, *Ireland's Trees*, 28–33.

86. Laurie, *Ogam,* 62–65.

87. Gregory, "Visions and Beliefs in the West of Ireland."

88. Culpeper, *The Complete Herbal,* 14.

89. Crow, *Native Plants, Native Healing.*

90. Wang et al., "Polygonatum Odoratum Polysaccharides."

91. Wood, *The Book of Herbal Wisdom,* 404.

92. Wood, *The Book of Herbal Wisdom,* 405.

93. Dictionary of Old English Plant Names, s.v. "Hlædder-Wyrt."

94. Wood, *The Book of Herbal Wisdom,* 404.

95. Woodland Essence, website.

96. Pendell and Snyder, *Pharmako Poeia.*

97. Culpeper, *The Complete Herbal,* 197.

98. Wood, *The Earthwise Herbal,* 112.

99. Iwersen, "Virgin Goddess."

100. Culpeper, *The Complete Herbal,* 123.

101. Wood, *The Earthwise Herbal,* 112–113.

Bibliography

Aaron, Elizabeth, Alicia Montgomery, Xinguo Ren, Stephen Guter, George Anderson, Ana M. Carneiro, Suma Jacob, et al. "Whole Blood Serotonin Levels and Platelet 5-HT2A Binding in Autism Spectrum Disorder." *Journal of Autism and Developmental Disorders* 49, no. 6 (2019): 2417–25. https://doi.org/10.1007/s10803-019-03989-z.

Anderson, Cora. *Fifty Years in the Feri Tradition*. Portland, Ore.: Harpy Books, 2010.

Anderson, Victor H., and Cora Anderson. *Etheric Anatomy: The Three Selves and Astral Travel*. Albany, Calif.: Acorn Guild Press, 2004.

Arie, Eran, Baruch Rosen, and Dvory Namdar. "Cannabis and Frankincense at the Judahite Shrine of Arad." *Tel Aviv* 47, no. 1 (2020): 5–28. https://doi.org/10.1080/03344355.2020.1732046.

Artisson, Robin. *An Carow Gwyn: Sorcery and the Ancient Fayerie Faith*. Bangor, Me.: Black Malkin Press, 2018.

———. *The Flaming Circle: A Reconstruction of the Old Ways of Britain and Ireland; A Modern Path-Guide to the Religious Practices and Spiritual Worldviews of the People of the Pre-Christian British Isles*. Los Angeles: Pendraig, 2008.

Bedi, Gillinder, David Hyman, and Harriet de Wit. "Is Ecstasy an 'Empathogen'? Effects of ±3,4-Methylenedioxymethamphetamine on Prosocial Feelings and Identification of Emotional States in Others." *Biological Psychiatry* 68, no. 12 (2010): 1134–40. https://doi.org/10.1016/j.biopsych.2010.08.003.

Benavidez, Cornelia. *Victor Anderson: An American Shaman*. Stafford, UK: Megalithica Books, 2017.

Bensky, Dan, Andrew Gamble, Steven Clavey, Stöger Erich, and Lilian Lai Bensky. *Chinese Herbal Medicine*. Seattle, Wash.: Eastland Press, 2015.

Bergamaschi, Mateus M., Regina Helena Queiroz, Marcos Hortes Chagas, Danielle Chaves de Oliveira, Bruno Spinosa De Martinis, Flávio Kapczinski, João Quevedo, et al. "Cannabidiol Reduces the Anxiety Induced by Simulated Public Speaking in Treatment-Naïve Social Phobia Patients." *Neuropsychopharmacology* 36, no. 6 (2011): 1219–26. https://doi .org/10.1038/npp.2011.6.

Blackie, Sharon. *If Women Rose Rooted: A Life-Changing Journey to Authenticity and Belonging.* Tewkesbury, Gloucestershire, UK: September Publishing, 2019.

Boericke, William. "Cannabis Indica, Hashish." In "The Tinctures," in *Boericke's Materia Medica,* 1901. Available online at Henriette's Herbal Homepage.

Bohbot, Véronique D., John J. Allen, Alain Dagher, Serge O. Dumoulin, Alan C. Evans, Michael Petrides, Miroslav Kalina, Katerina Stepankova, and Lynn Nadel. "Role of the Parahippocampal Cortex in Memory for the Configuration but Not the Identity of Objects: Converging Evidence from Patients with Selective Thermal Lesions and fMRI." *Frontiers in Human Neuroscience* 9 (2015). https://doi.org/10.3389/fnhum.2015.00431.

Bossong, Matthijs G., Hendrika H. van Hell, Chris D. Schubart, Wesley van Saane, Tabitha A. Iseger, Gerry Jager, Matthias J. P. van Osch, et al. "Acute Effects of Δ9-Tetrahydrocannabinol (THC) on Resting State Brain Function and Their Modulation by COMT Genotype." *European Neuropsychopharmacology* 29, no. 6 (2019): 766–76. https://doi .org/10.1016/j.euroneuro.2019.03.010.

Bromwich, Jonah E. "The Capital That Ate Wellness Is Going to Eat Your Mushrooms." *New York Times,* February 28, 2020.

Buhner, Stephen Harrod. *Plant Intelligence and the Imaginal Realm: Beyond the Doors of Perception into the Dreaming Earth*. Rochester, Vt.: Bear & Co., 2014.

———. "SARS-CoV-2 Protocol." Stephen Harrod Buhner website, August 20, 2022.

———. *The Secret Teachings of Plants: The Intelligence of the Heart in the Direct Perception of Nature*. Rochester, Vt.: Bear & Co., 2004.

———. *Vital Man: Natural Health Care for Men at Midlife*. New York: Avery, 2003.

Burch, Michael R., trans. "The Song of Amergin." Song of Amergin: Modern English Translations, The Hypertexts (website).

Camus, Albert. *Personal Writings*. New York: Vintage, 2020.

Carhart-Harris, Robin L., Leor Roseman, Mark Bolstridge, Lysia Demetriou, J. Nienke Pannekoek, Matthew B. Wall, Mark Tanner, et al. "Psilocybin for Treatment-Resistant Depression: Fmri-Measured Brain Mechanisms." *Scientific Reports* 7, no. 1 (2017). https://doi.org/10.1038/s41598-017-13282-7.

Carhart-Harris, Robin L., Suresh Muthukumaraswamy, Leor Roseman, Mendel Kaelen, Wouter Droog, Kevin Murphy, Enzo Tagliazucchi, et al. "Neural Correlates of the LSD Experience Revealed by Multimodal Neuroimaging." *Proceedings of the National Academy of Sciences* 113, no. 17 (2016): 4853–58. https://doi.org/10.1073/pnas.1518377113.

Child, Francis James. "37A: Thomas Rymer." In vol. 1 of *The English and Scottish Popular Ballads*. 10 vols. New York: Houghton Mifflin, 1882–1898. Available online at Internet Sacred Text Archive.

Cockayne, Thomas Oswald. *Leechdoms, Wortcunning and Starcraft in Early England: Being a Collection of Documents, for the Most Part Never before Printed, Illustrating the History of Science in This Country before the Norman Conquest*. London, 1864.

Cook, William H. "Cimicifuga Racemosa. Black Cohosh, Rattleroot." In *The Physio-Medical Dispensatory: A Treatise on Therapeutics*. London, 1869. Available online at Henriette's Herbal Homepage.

———. "Symplocarpus Foetidus. Skunk Cabbage." In *The Physio-Medical Dispensatory: A Treatise on Therapeutics*. London, 1869. Available online at Henriette's Herbal Homepage.

Cox, Christine L., Lucina Q. Uddin, Adriana Di Martino, F. Xavier Castellanos, Michael P. Milham, and Clare Kelly. "The Balance between Feeling and Knowing: Affective and Cognitive Empathy Are Reflected in the Brain's Intrinsic Functional Dynamics." *Social Cognitive and Affective Neuroscience* 7, no. 6 (2011): 727–37. https://doi.org/10.1093/scan/nsr051.

Crippa, José Alexandre, Antonio Waldo Zuardi, Griselda E Garrido, Lauro Wichert-Ana, Ricardo Guarnieri, Lucas Ferrari, Paulo M. Azevedo-Marques, Jaime Eduardo Hallak, Philip K. McGuire, and Geraldo Filho Busatto. "Effects of Cannabidiol (CBD) on Regional Cerebral Blood Flow." *Neuropsychopharmacology* 29, no. 2 (2003): 417–26. https://doi.org/10.1038/sj.npp.1300340.

Crow, Tis Mal. *Native Plants, Native Healing: Traditional Muskogee Way.* Summertown, Tenn.: Native Voices, 2001.

Crowley, Aleister. *Magick in Theory and Practice.* Oxfordshire, UK: 1929.

Culpeper, Nicholas. *The Complete Herbal.* London: Thomas Kelly, 1835. Available online at Project Gutenberg.

Daimler, Morgan. *Manannán Mac Lir: Meeting the Celtic God of Wave and Wonder.* Winchester, UK: Moon Books, 2019.

———.*The Morrigan: Meeting the Great Queens.* Winchester, UK: Moon Books, 2014.

———. *Pagan Portals: Brigid: Meeting the Celtic Goddess of Poetry, Forge, and Healing Well.* Winchester, UK: Moon Books, 2016.

Dharmananda, Subhuti. "Kidney Essence and the Human Body: An Exploration of Chinese Embryology." Institute for Traditional Medicine (website).

Di Marzo, Vincenzo, and Fabiana Piscitelli. "The Endocannabinoid System and Its Modulation by Phytocannabinoids." *Neurotherapeutics* 12, no. 4 (2015): 692–98. https://doi.org/10.1007/s13311-015-0374-6.

Dimech, Alkistis. "Dynamics of the Occulted Body." In *The Brazen Vessel.* Cornwall, UK: Scarlet Imprint, 2019.

di Tomaso, Emmanuelle, Massimiliano Beltramo, and Daniele Piomelli. "Brain Cannabinoids in Chocolate." *Nature* 382, no. 6593 (1996): 677–78. https://doi.org/10.1038/382677a0.

Dōgen, Eihei. *Moon in a Dewdrop: Writings of Zen Master Dōgen.* Edited by Kazuaki Tanahashi. San Francisco: North Point Press, 1995.

Duvall, Chris S. "A Brief Agricultural History of Cannabis in Africa, from Prehistory to Canna-Colony." *EchoGéo*, no. 48 (2019). https://doi.org/10.4000/echogeo.17599.

Edwards, Gail Faith. *Opening Our Wild Hearts to the Healing Herbs.* Woodstock, N.Y.: Ash Tree, 2000.

Ellingwood, Finley, and John Uri Lloyd. *American Materia Medica, Therapeutics and Pharmacognosy.* Chicago: Ellingwood's Theraputist, 1915. Available online at Henriette's Herbal Homepage.

Federici, Silvia. "In Praise of the Dancing Body." *Gods & Radicals*, August 21, 2016.

Felter, Harvey Wickes, and John Uri Lloyd. "Dracontium.—Skunk-Cabbage." In *King's American Dispensatory.* Cincinnati: Ohio Valley, 1898. Available online at Henriette's Herbal Homepage.

Foucault, Michel. *The Birth of the Clinic: An Archaeology of Medical Perception.* London: Routledge, 2010.

Frances, Deborah. Crataegus: "Mental and Emotional Indications." North American Institute of Medical Herbalism, Inc. medherb.com.

Frank, Adam, David Grinspoon, and Sara Walker. "Intelligence as a Planetary Scale Process." *International Journal of Astrobiology* 21, no. 2 (2022): 47–61. https://doi.org/10.1017/s147355042100029x.

Gantz, Jeffrey. *Early Irish Myths and Sagas*. London: Penguin Books, 1988.

Gregory, Lady Augusta. "Visions and Beliefs in the West of Ireland Index." *Visions and Beliefs in the West of Ireland*. Available at Sacred Texts online.

Gwynn, Edward, trans. *The Metrical Dindshenchas*. Commentary by Edward Gwynn. Dublin: Hodges, Figgis, 1903. Available online at Corpus of Electronic Texts Edition.

Hardin, Kiva Rose. "Alder." Enchanter's Green. enchantersgreen.com.

Heaney, Seamus. *Sweeney Astray*. London: Faber and Faber, 2001.

———. Door in the Dark. London: Faber and Faber, 1972.

Hill, M. N., S. Patel, P. Campolongo, J. G. Tasker, C. T. Wotjak, and J. S. Bains. "Functional Interactions between Stress and the Endocannabinoid System: From Synaptic Signaling to Behavioral Output." *Journal of Neuroscience* 30, no. 45 (2010): 14980–86. https://doi.org/10.1523/jneurosci.4283-10.2010.

Holze, Friederike, Patrick Vizeli, Felix Müller, Laura Ley, Raoul Duerig, Nimmy Varghese, Anne Eckert, Stefan Borgwardt, and Matthias E. Liechti. "Distinct Acute Effects of LSD, MDMA, and D-Amphetamine in Healthy Subjects." *Neuropsychopharmacology* 45, no. 3 (2019): 462–71. https://doi.org/10.1038/s41386-019-0569-3.

Iwersen, Julia. "Virgin Goddess." *Encyclopedia of Religion*. Encyclopedia.com, January 2005.

Jensen, Derrick. *Listening to the Land: Conversations about Nature, Culture, and Eros*. White River Junction, Vt: Chelsea Green, 2004.

Jobst, Beatrice M., Selen Atasoy, Adrián Ponce-Alvarez, Ana Sanjuán, Leor Roseman, Mendel Kaelen, Robin Carhart-Harris, Morten L. Kringelbach, and Gustavo Deco. "Increased Sensitivity to Strong Perturbations in a Whole-Brain Model of LSD." *NeuroImage* 230 (2021): 117809. https://doi.org/10.1016/j.neuroimage.2021.117809.

Kearney, Peadar. "Bold Fenian Men." Available online at All Poetry.

Kimmerer, Robin Wall. *Braiding Sweetgrass: Indigenous Wisdom, Scientific Knowledge and the Teachings of Plants*. New York: Penguin Books, 2020.

Ko, G. D., S. L. Bober, S. Mindra, and J. M. Moreau. "Medical Cannabis: The Canadian Perspective." *Journal of Pain Research* 9 (2016): 735–44. https://doi.org/10.2147/JPR.S98182.

Kozela, Ewa, Maciej Pietr, Ana Juknat, Neta Rimmerman, Rivka Levy, and Zvi Vogel. "Cannabinoids Δ9-Tetrahydrocannabinol and Cannabidiol Differentially Inhibit the Lipopolysaccharide-Activated NF-KB and Interferon-β/Stat Proinflammatory Pathways in BV-2 Microglial Cells." *Journal of Biological Chemistry* 285, no. 3 (2010): 1616–26. https://doi.org/10.1074/jbc.m109.069294.

"Kuhn, Maggie." Available online at National Women's Hall of Fame.

Kvilhaug, Maria. *The Seed of Yggdrasill*. Elliot Lake, Ontario: Three Little Sisters, 2020.

Laurie, Erynn Rowan. "The Cauldron of Poesy." The Preserving Shrine: Eryn Rowan Laurie, 2010 (website).

———. *Ogam: Weaving Word Wisdom*. Stafford, UK: Megalithica Books, 2007.

Laurie, Erynn Rowan, and Timothy White. "Speckled Snake, Brother of Birch: Amanita Muscaria Motifs in Celtic Legends." *Shaman's Drum* 44 (1997).

Leary, Timothy. *Neuropolitique*. With Robert Anton Wilson, and George A. Koopman. Scottsdale, Ariz.: New Falcon Press, 2006. First published 1977 as *Neuropolitics: The Sociobiology of Human Metamorphosis*.

Lee, Jonathan L., Leandro J. Bertoglio, Francisco S. Guimarães, and Carl W. Stevenson. "Cannabidiol Regulation of Emotion and Emotional Memory Processing: Relevance for Treating Anxiety-Related and Substance Abuse Disorders." *British Journal of Pharmacology* 174, no. 19 (2017): 3242–56. https://doi.org/10.1111/bph.13724.

Lenihan, Edmund, and Carolyn Eve Green. *Meeting the Other Crowd: The Fairy Stories of Hidden Ireland*. New York: Jeremy P. Tarcher/Putnam, 2004.

Leopold, Aldo, and Luna B. Leopold. *Round River: From the Journals of Aldo Leopold*. Oxford: Oxford University Press, 1993.

Lifton, Robert Jay, and Richard A. Falk. *Indefensible Weapons: The Political and Psychological Case against Nuclearism*. New York: Basic Books, 1991.

Lorca, Federico Garcia. "Theory and Play of the Duende." Translated by A. S. Kilne. Poetry in Translation (website), 2007.

Loughlin, Annie. "Gods and Spirits." Tairis: A Gaelic Polytheist Website, 2006–2018.

Lyons, Taylor, and Robin L. Carhart-Harris. "Increased Nature Relatedness and Decreased Authoritarian Political Views after Psilocybin for Treatment-

Resistant Depression." *Journal of Psychopharmacology* 32, no. 7 (2018): 811–19. https://doi.org/10.1177/0269881117748902.

Mac Coitir, Niall. *Ireland's Trees: Myths, Legends and Folklore*. Cork, Ireland: Collins Press, 2016.

———. *Ireland's Wild Plants: Myths, Legends and Folklore*. Cork, Ireland: Collins Press, 2017

Mac Coitir, Niall, and Gordon D'Arcy. *Ireland's Animals: Myths, Legends and Folklore*. Cork, Ireland: Collins Press, 2015.

Macy, Joanna, and Molly Young Brown. *Coming Back to Life: The Updated Guide to The Work That Reconnects*. Gabriola Island, BC: New Society, 2014.

Magan, Manchán. *Thirty-Two Words for Field: Lost Words of the Irish Landscape*. Dublin: Gill Books, 2020.

Mann, Jeremy. "How San Francisco's HIV/AIDS Warriors Paved the Way for Today's Cannabis Gold Rush." *San Francisco Chronicle*, May 7, 2019.

Masé, Guido. *The Wild Medicine Solution: Healing with Aromatic, Bitter, and Tonic Plants*. Rochester, Vt.: Healing Arts Press, 2013.

mcdonald, jim. "Herbal Properties and Actions." jim mcdonald Herbalist, Herbcraft.org.

Moriarty, John. *Dreamtime*. Dublin: Lilliput Press, 2009.

———. *Invoking Ireland: Ailiu Iath n-hErend*. Dublin: Lilliput Press, 2006.

———. "Seeking to Walk Beautifully on the Earth." YouTube video, 2:58:51, August 2, 2020. Posted by Francis Cassidy.

Murphy, Anthony. *Finn and the Salmon of Knowledge: Mythology, Toponymy and Cosmology*. Drogheda: Mythical Ireland, 2021.

Naess, Arne. "Self-Realization: An Ecological Approach to Being in the World." In *The Selected Works of Arne Naess*. Berlin: Springer, 2005

Nayak, Sandeep M., and Roland R. Griffiths. "A Single Belief-Changing Psychedelic Experience Is Associated with Increased Attribution of Consciousness to Living and Non-Living Entities." *Frontiers in Psychology* 13 (2022). https://doi.org/10.3389/fpsyg.2022.852248.

O'Donoghue, Seán Padraig. *Courting the Wild Queen*. Luxembourg: Ritona Press, 2022.

Pellati, Federica, Vittoria Borgonetti, Virginia Brighenti, Marco Biagi, Stefania Benvenuti, and Lorenzo Corsi. "*Cannabis Sativa* L. and Nonpsychoactive Cannabinoids: Their Chemistry and Role against Oxidative Stress, Inflammation, and Cancer." *BioMed Research International* 2018 (2018): 1–15. https://doi.org/10.1155/2018/1691428.

Pendell, Dale. *Pharmako Dynamis: Stimulating Plants, Potions, and Herbcraft: Excitantia and Empathogenica*. Berkeley, Calif.: North Atlantic Books, 2009.

———. *Pharmako Gnosis: Plant Teachers and the Poison Path*. Berkeley, Calif.: North Atlantic Books, 2009.

Pendell, Dale, and Gary Snyder. *Pharmako Poeia: Plant Powers, Poisons, and Herbcraft*. Berkeley, Calif.: North Atlantic Books, 2010.

Pert, Candace B. *Molecules of Emotion: Why You Feel the Way You Feel*. New York: Scribner, 2003.

Philpott, Holly T., Melissa O'Brien, and Jason J. McDougall. "Attenuation of Early Phase Inflammation by Cannabidiol Prevents Pain and Nerve Damage in Rat Osteoarthritis." *Pain* 158, no. 12 (2017): 2442–51. https://doi.org/10.1097/j.pain.0000000000001052.

Preller, Katrin H., Leonhard Schilbach, Thomas Pokorny, Jan Flemming, Erich Seifritz, and Franz X. Vollenweider. "Role of the 5-HT2a Receptor in Self- and Other-Initiated Social Interaction in Lysergic Acid Diethylamide-Induced States: A Pharmacological Fmri Study." *Journal of Neuroscience* 38, no. 14 (2018): 3603–11. https://doi.org/10.1523/jneurosci.1939-17.2018.

Prud'homme, Mélissa, Romulus Cata, and Didier Jutras-Aswad. "Cannabidiol as an Intervention for Addictive Behaviors: A Systematic Review of the Evidence." *Substance Abuse: Research and Treatment* 9 (2015). https://doi.org/10.4137/sart.s25081.

Ramos, Valeriano. "The Concepts of Ideology, Hegemony, and Organic Intellectuals in Gramsci's Marxism." *Theoretical Review*, no. 27 (March–April 1982).

Reich, Wilhelm. *Ether, God, Devil and Cosmic Superimposition*. New York: Farrar, Straus and Giroux, 1973.

———. *The Function of the Orgasm: Sex-Economic Problems of Biological Energy*. New York: Pocket Books, 1978.

———. *The Mass Psychology of Fascism*. London: Souvenir Press, 2018.

Ren, Meng, Zihua Tang, Xinhua Wu, Robert Spengler, Hongen Jiang, Yimin Yang, and Nicole Boivin. "The Origins of Cannabis Smoking: Chemical Residue Evidence from the First Millennium BCE in the Pamirs." *Science Advances* 5, no. 6 (2019). https://doi.org/10.1126/sciadv.aaw1391.

Roseman, Leor, David J. Nutt, and Robin L. Carhart-Harris. "Quality of Acute Psychedelic Experience Predicts Therapeutic Efficacy of Psilocybin for Treatment-Resistant Depression." *Frontiers in Pharmacology* 8 (2018). https://doi.org/10.3389/fphar.2017.00974.

Ross, Stephen, Anthony Bossis, Jeffrey Guss, Gabrielle Agin-Liebes, Tara Malone, Barry Cohen, Sarah E. Mennenga, et al. "Rapid and Sustained Symptom Reduction Following Psilocybin Treatment for Anxiety and Depression in Patients with Life-Threatening Cancer: A Randomized Controlled Trial." *Journal of Psychopharmacology* 30, no. 12 (2016): 1165–80. https://doi .org/10.1177/0269881116675512.

Russo, Ethan. "Cannabinoids in the Management of Difficult to Treat Pain." *Therapeutics and Clinical Risk Management* 4 (2008): 245–59. https://doi .org/10.2147/tcrm.s1928.

———. "Clinical Endocannabinoid Deficiency Reconsidered: Current Research Supports the Theory in Migraine, Fibromyalgia, Irritable Bowel, and Other Treatment-Resistant Syndromes." *Cannabis and Cannabinoid Research* 1, no. 1 (2016): 154–65. https://doi.org/10.1089/can.2016.0009.

———. "Taming THC: Potential Cannabis Synergy and Phytocannabinoid-Terpenoid Entourage Effects." *British Journal of Pharmacology* 163, no. 7 (2011): 1344–64. https://doi.org/10.1111/j.1476-5381.2011.01238.x.

Savarese, Ralph. "I Object: Autism, Empathy, and the Trope of Personification." YouTube video, 53:55, Emory University, March 3, 2014.

Scahill, Lawrence, and George M. Anderson. "Is Ecstasy an Empathogen?" *Biological Psychiatry* 68, no. 12 (2010): 1082–83. https://doi.org/10.1016/j .biopsych.2010.10.020.

Scallon, Dana Rosemary. "Lady of Knock," 1981. Available at "Collection of Irish Song Lyrics," Donal O'Shaughnessy Irish Songs, 2011.

Schiffman, Richard. "Psilocybin: A Journey beyond the Fear of Death?" *Scientific American*, December 1, 2016.

Schulke, Daniel A. *Viridarium Umbris: The Pleasure Garden of Shadows.* Chelmsford, UK: Xoanon, 2005.

Senst, Laura, and Jaideep Bains. "Neuromodulators, Stress and Plasticity: A Role for Endocannabinoid Signalling." *Journal of Experimental Biology* 217, no. 1 (2014): 102–8. https://doi.org/10.1242/jeb.089730.

Shalev, Ido, and Florina Uzefovsky. "Empathic Disequilibrium in Two Different Measures of Empathy Predicts Autism Traits in Neurotypical Population." *Molecular Autism* 11, no. 1 (2020). https://doi.org/10.1186/ s13229-020-00362-1.

Shannon, S., and J. Opihla-Lehman "Effectiveness of Cannabidiol Oil for Pediatric Anxiety and Insomnia as Part of Posttraumatic Stress Disorder: A Case Report." *Permanente Journal*, 2019. https://doi.org/10.7812/TPP/16-005.

Sheldrake, Merlin. *Entangled Life: How Fungi Make Our Worlds, Change Our Minds and Shape Our Futures.* London: Vintage, 2021.

Snyder, Gary. *A Place in Space: Ethics, Aesthetics, and Watersheds; New and Selected Prose.* Berkeley, Calif.: Counterpoint, 2008.

Sulak, Dustin. "How to Stimulate the Endocannabinoid System without Cannabis." *Leafly,* July 28, 2020.

Tagliazucchi, Enzo, Leor Roseman, Mendel Kaelen, Csaba Orban, Suresh D. Muthukumaraswamy, Kevin Murphy, Helmut Laufs, et al. "Increased Global Functional Connectivity Correlates with LSD-Induced Ego Dissolution." *Current Biology* 26, no. 8 (2016): 1043–50. https://doi .org/10.1016/j.cub.2016.02.010.

Tauring, Kari. *Runes: A Deeper Journey.* LULU COM, 2018.

Temple, Emily November. "Here It Is! Alice B. Toklas's Recipe for Hash Brownies." Literary Hub (website), April 1, 2019.

Thoreau, Henry David. "'Wild Apples: The History of the Apple-Tree." *Atlantic,* November 1862.

Tozzi, Paolo. "Does Fascia Hold Memories?" *Journal of Bodywork and Movement Therapies* 18, no. 2 (2014): 259–65. https://doi.org/10.1016/j .jbmt.2013.11.010.

Vučković, Sonja, Dragana Srebro, Katarina Savić Vujović, Čedomir Vučetić, and Milica Prostran. "Cannabinoids and Pain: New Insights from Old Molecules." *Frontiers in Pharmacology* 9 (2018). https://doi.org/10.3389/ fphar.2018.01259.

Walker, Nick. "Throw Away the Master's Tools: Liberating Ourselves from the Pathology Paradigm." In *Loud Hands: Autistic People, Speaking,* 225–37. Edited by Julia Bascom. Washington, D.C.: Autistic Press, 2012.

———. "What Is Autism?" Neuroqueer: The Writings of Dr. Nick Walker (website), 2014.

Wang, Yan, Yanquan Fei, Lirui Liu, Yunhua Xiao, Yilin Pang, Jinhe Kang, and Zheng Wang. "*Polygonatum Odoratum* Polysaccharides Modulate Gut Microbiota and Mitigate Experimentally Induced Obesity in Rats." *International Journal of Molecular Sciences* 19, no. 11 (2018): 3587. https:// doi.org/10.3390/ijms19113587.

Hedley, Gil. "The Way We Are Designed: A Conversation with Gil Hedley, PhD." Interview by Jennifer Walters. *Acupuncture Today,* April 2015.

Weschler, Lawrence. "A Rare, Personal Look at Oliver Sacks's Early Career." *Vanity Fair,* April 28, 2015.

Weizman, Libat, Lior Dayan, Silviu Brill, Hadas Nahman-Averbuch, Talma Hendler, Giris Jacob, and Haggai Sharon. "Cannabis Analgesia in Chronic Neuropathic Pain Is Associated with Altered Brain Connectivity." *Neurology* 91, no. 14 (2018). https://doi.org/10.1212/wnl.0000000000006293.

Wilde, Lady Jane Francesca. *Ancient Legends, Mystic Charms, and Superstitions of Ireland.* London: Chatto & Windus, 1919. Available online at Project Gutenberg.

Wilson, Peter Lamborn. *Ploughing the Clouds: The Search for Irish Soma.* San Francisco: City Lights, 1999.

Wood, Matthew. *The Book of Herbal Wisdom: Using Plants as Medicine.* Berkeley, Calif.: North Atlantic Books, 1998.

———. *Vitalism: The History of Herbalism, Homeopathy and Flower Essences.* Berkeley, Calif.: North Atlantic Books, 2000.

———. *The Earthwise Herbal: A Complete Guide to New World Medicinal Plants.* Berkeley, Calif.: North Atlantic Books, 2009.

———. *The Earthwise Herbal: A Complete Guide to Old World Medicinal Plants.* Berkeley, Calif.: North Atlantic Books, 2008.

Yeats, William Butler. "The Song of Wandering Aengus." Poetry Foundation (website). Accessed December 6, 2023.

Yirmiya, Raz, Neta Rimmerman, and Ronen Reshef. "Depression as a Microglial Disease." *Trends in Neurosciences* 38, no. 10 (2015): 637–58. https://doi.org/10.1016/j.tins.2015.08.001.

Zuardi, Antonio Waldo. "History of Cannabis as a Medicine: A Review." *Revista Brasileira de Psiquiatria* 28, no. 2 (2006): 153–57. https://doi.org/10.1590/s1516-44462006000200015.

Index

About the Author

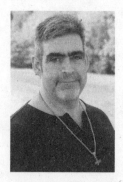

Seán Pádraig O'Donoghue is an herbalist, teacher, and Earth poet living in western Maine. He is an initiated priest of the Feri and Crossroads traditions. Prior to becoming an herbalist, Seán was a political organizer in movements for peace, human rights, and global economic justice and a freelance journalist documenting the human and ecological impacts of U.S. policies in Latin America.

Seán grew up near Boston, a short distance from where his great-grandparents first landed when they arrived from Ireland. Since childhood, he has been an avid student of Irish history and folklore. He graduated from Dartmouth College in 1996 with a degree in English literature and creative writing.